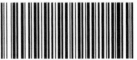

ALPHA LIPOIC ACID

Nature's Ultimate Antioxidant

BOOK YOUR PLACE ON OUR WEBSITE AND MAKE THE READING CONNECTION!

We've created a customized website just for our very special readers, where you can get the inside scoop on everything that's going on with Zebra, Pinnacle and Kensington books.

When you come online, you'll have the exciting opportunity to:

- View covers of upcoming books

- Read sample chapters

- Learn about our future publishing schedule (listed by publication month *and author*)

- Find out when your favorite authors will be visiting a city near you

- Search for and order backlist books from our online catalog

- Check out author bios and background information

- Send e-mail to your favorite authors

- Meet the Kensington staff online

- Join us in weekly chats with authors, readers and other guests

- Get writing guidelines

- AND MUCH MORE!

Visit our website at
http://www.kensingtonbooks.com

ALPHA LIPOIC ACID

Nature's Ultimate Antioxidant

Allan E. Sosin, M.D., Medical Director,
Whitaker Wellness Institute,
and Beth M. Ley Jacobs, Ph.D.

Foreword by Julian Whitaker, M.D.

Kensington Books
http://www.kensingtonbooks.com

This publication and product is designed to provide accurate and authoritative information with regard to the subject matter covered. The purchase of this publication does not create a doctor-patient relationship between the purchaser and the author, nor should the information contained in this book be considered specific medical advice with respect to a specific patient and/or a specific condition. In the event the purchaser desires to obtain specific medical advice or other information concerning a specific person, condition, or situation, the services of a competent professional should be sought.

The author and publisher specifically disclaim any liability, loss, or risk, personal or otherwise, that is or may be incurred as a consequence, directly or indirectly, of the use and application of any of the information contained in this book.

KENSINGTON BOOKS are published by

Kensington Publishing Corp.
850 Third Avenue
New York, NY 10022

Copyright © 1998 by Allan E. Sosin and Beth M. Ley Jacobs

Credits:

Artwork: Stephanie Scott

Technical Assistance:
  Dr. Lester Packer, University of California, Berkeley
  Sid Shastri, Jarrow Formulas, Los Angeles

Kensington and the K logo Reg. U.S. Pat. & TM Off.

First Printing: December, 1998
10 9 8 7 6 5 4 3 2 1

Printed in the United States of America

Contents

Foreword

by Julian Whitaker, M.D.

Free radical damage has been established as a primary
contributor to a wide range of degenerative diseases—and the aging process itself. Antioxidants,
such as vitamin C, vitamin E, vitamin A, and beta-
carotene quench free radicals and are among the
most powerful nutrients for the maintenance of optimal health.

In recent years a new generation of antioxidants
have hit the supplement shelves, and the best and
brightest of them is Alpha Lipoic Acid. This versatile
antioxidant has the unique ability to neutralize both
water- and fat-soluble free radicals as well as rejuve-
nate other antioxidants back into their active, protective forms. Alpha Lipoic Acid is also essential for
energy production and the metabolism of sugar.

I first learned about Alpha Lipoic Acid several
years ago from German researchers studying its
effects on diabetes. The result of their research were
so astounding, particularly in improving the compli-

cations of diabetes, that I immediately began using it in my medical practice. Since that time, Alpha Lipoic Acid has become an indispensable therapeutic tool at Whitaker Wellness Institute. In addition to helping diabetic patients' peripheral neuropathy and blood sugar control, it is an invaluable adjunct in the treatment of liver disorders, cardiovascular disease, AIDS, and eye problems.

My colleague, Allan Sosin, M.D., and Beth Ley Jacobs, Ph.D., have done a commendable job sorting out the research on this very complex substance. I would love to see this book read by each and every physician in this country. My more realistic hope, however, is that enough interest will be generated by this book and the people who read it that Alpha Lipoic Acid will emerge from obscurity into the hands of people who will reap its significant benefits.

Introduction

I want you to know why I am the kind of doctor I am. I see the main problem with medicine today in the kind of treatment given by doctors and accepted by patients. Quite simply, patients have become secondary to their diseases. Physicians usually concentrate on labeling the disease and finding a drug or an operation that treats the disease. The person, with his or her dreams, debts, obligations and fears, becomes a bystander in the conflict between the affliction and the doctor(s).

Within a patient's life and mind, however, lie keys to the unfolding of illness. When a condition will not yield to usual treatments, the physician needs to look again to the patient for other information toward a different course of action.

Over and over again have I seen the individual, in this case usually male, with hypertension and diabetes, who was started on a diuretic for high blood pressure which didn't work, so then Lopressor, Cardizem, and Cozaar were added. For the diabetes he gets Micronase, then Glucophage, and then insulin. He finally comes to me weighing 230 pounds, still with high blood pressure, complains of memory loss and fatigue, and hasn't had an erection in six months.

Why isn't the multidrug regimen working?

It turns out that he drinks twelve cups of coffee a day, loves orange juice for breakfast, and works too many hours to have any time left for exercise, even half an hour for walking. Beyond this, there is a host of personal issues. Perhaps his wife's mother has moved in, his son wants to drop out of school, unpaid bills are mounting up, and gas pains keep him awake at night.

At Whitaker Wellness Institute we examine *all* this information. Obtaining an accurate nutritional history is crucial as well. Knowledge of family circumstances, work stresses, environmental exposures, personal attitudes and intentions, and other reasons for depression and hopelessness is important for making an *informed diagnosis*.

It is the kind of diagnosis that physicians need to make and must make today as a matter of course.

I joined Dr. Julian Whitaker in his clinic at 4321 Birch Street, Newport Beach, California, two years ago. People come to this clinic from across the country and from other countries, hoping to improve their health with nondrug, nonsurgical methods, and because they know that at Whitaker they will receive exceptional care.

Daily we see patients with heart disease, diabetes

mellitus, and hypertension, and many others with chronic fatigue, memory loss, arthritis, allergic conditions, depression, gastrointestinal disturbances, and a general failure to thrive. We have a full-time nutritionist experienced in the application of macrobiotics, low glycemic index diets, milk and gluten-free diets, and other specialized nutritional programs. We work with chiropractors, message therapists, acupuncturists, exercise physiologists and therapists, reflexologists, herbalists, and counselors.

Our regimens of vitamin, mineral, hormonal, metabolic, and herbal therapies are extensive and constantly growing. When properly applied, these are safe and effective therapies. They do not produce the cumulative and collaborative toxicities that commonly occur from the kinds of multidrug therapies too quickly and too carelessly given today.

Alpha Lipoic Acid was added to our list of nutritional substances more than a year ago. We use it routinely in the management of patients with diabetes mellitus, especially those with evidence of end organ damage such as proliferative retinopathy, macular degeneration, or peripheral neuropathy. We use it in the treatment of liver diseases, eye diseases, neurological problems, cardiac diseases, and any other condition where free radical damage is considered contributory.

We do not recommend Alpha Lipoic Acid alone, but always in conjunction with other agents in order to provide excellent, coordinated benefits.

In nature things do not stand alone. Chemicals found in plants, now called "phytonutrients," are present in the plant to protect it from various environmental stresses. We know that many of these chemicals can have a similar protective effect on our health.

In this book we will explain how Alpha Lipoic Acid, used in conjunction with other supplements in a comprehensive program, can improve a variety of medical conditions. I have recommended it to hundreds of patients. I am in good health and take 150 mg of Alpha Lipoic Acid daily to stay that way.

Allan E. Sosin

CHAPTER 1

Alpha Lipoic Acid

Alpha Lipoic Acid, also known as Thioctic Acid, is a vitamin-like antioxidant which is produced naturally in the body. It is not considered a vitamin because presumably either the body can produce it in sufficient amounts or it is acquired in sufficient quantities from food. Many situations, however, can lead to deficiency. What is especially exciting is its use as a dietary supplement. Taken orally, for instance, Alpha Lipoic Acid exerts benefits certainly beyond its normal roles in the body and is capable of producing tremendous results.

We have known about the existence of Alpha Lipoic Acid since the 1930s when a so-called "potato growth factor" was discovered as necessary for the growth of certain bacteria. In 1957, the compound was extracted and formally identified as Alpha Lipoic Acid.

By 1998, of course, the unique properties of Alpha Lipoic Acid have been clearly demonstrated and its popularity is growing rapidly. At the same time, we as a population have become more and more aware of the huge impact free radicals and free radical damage have upon our state of health and rate of aging.

Alpha Lipoic Acid holds promise as a free radical protectant for our cells as it is the only antioxidant which is both fat- and water-soluble. This means that Alpha Lipoic Acid is easily absorbed and transported across cell membranes, offering us protection against free radical damage both inside and outside the cell. This is unlike many other antioxidants which provide extracellular protection only.

Cofactor for Energy Production

Under normal conditions, Alpha Lipoic Acid functions as a cofactor for a number of vital enzymes responsible for digesting and metabolizing our food to its chemical energy (ATP) form.

> Dr. Lester Packer, one of the world's leading researchers in the area of antioxidants and Alpha Lipoic Acid, stated in a press release that *"Alpha Lipoic Acid could have far-reaching consequences in the search for prevention and therapy of chronic degenerative diseases such as diabetes and cardiovascular disease. And because it is the only antioxidant that can get easily get into the brain, it could be useful in preventing damage from a stroke."*

Alpha Lipoic Acid is needed to produce energy at the cellular level.

Naturally Found in Foods We Eat Every Day

Outside the body, Alpha Lipoic Acid is found in the leaves of plants containing mitochondria and in nonphotosynthetic plant tissues, such as potatoes, spinach, broccoli, tomatoes, carrots, yams, and sweet potatoes. Red meat, especially liver and heart, is also a rich source of naturally occurring Alpha Lipoic Acid.

Therapeutic Applications

Alpha Lipoic Acid has been used throughout Europe to treat and prevent complications associated with diabetes including neuropathy, macular degeneration, and cataracts. More specific and varied therapeutic applications are noted below:

- Diabetes mellitus, for control of blood sugar and prevention and treatment of diabetic complications, including retinopathy, neuropathy, renal disease, and atherosclerosis.
- Liver diseases, including those caused by toxins, viruses such as hepatitis A, B, and C; alcohol; and drugs.
- Eye diseases, including macular degeneration and cataracts.
- Peripheral neuropathy.
- Neurologic diseases, including multiple sclerosis, stroke, and spinal cord injuries.
- Coronary artery disease and congestive heart failure.
- Vascular protective agent—such as for varicose

veins, leg cramps, easy bruising from capillary brittleness, and hemorrhoids.
- Reduction of the negative effects of inflammatory disorders such as asthma, allergies, sinusitis, hives, arthritis, etc.
- Cancer protection—protecting damage from radical agents to DNA, cellular membranes, lipids, proteins, etc.
- Inhibiting the replication of HIV (the virus associated with AIDS) and other viruses.
- Removal of heavy metals from the body.
- Prevention of radiation damage (internal and external) such as from the sun or X-rays, etc.
- Protection from premature aging.
- Prevention and relief of dry skin.
- Prevention and relief of sexual dysfunction in some males.
- In general, improvement of circulation, such as experienced by cold hands, cold feet, cold nose, etc.
- Speeds tissue healing and injury repair.
- For general health and maintenance of ideal antioxidant status in the body, in combination with other antioxidants including vitamin C, vitamin E, coenzyme Q-10, and pycnogenol.

In any situation in the body involving free radicals—including cancer, heart disease, and problems involving inflammation such as arthritis, asthma, allergies, and wounds such as sprains or lacerations—Alpha Lipoic Acid can be of great benefit. These situations are discussed in some detail later in this book.

CHAPTER 2

Free Radicals and Antioxidants

Just 10 or 15 years ago, free radicals were little known to most of us. Researchers now tell us that free radical damage throughout the body is a major cause of aging and age-associated disease.

Why is this so? The answer returns us to the free radical itself. A free radical is an unstable, incomplete molecule. It is incomplete because it is missing an electron which exists in pairs in stable molecules. Free radicals are unstable because they "steal" an electron from another molecule, and thereby create another free radical. This new free radical then duplicates the process, resulting in a chain reaction of events, which can ultimately damage the body.

Oxidation and Reduction (Redox)

Oxidation occurs when a molecule loses an electron. *Reduction* occurs when a molecule gains an elec-

How Antioxidants Stop Free Radicals

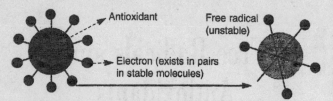

Figure 1—How Antioxidants Stop Free Radicals.

tron. Reducing power defines the ability of a compound to donate an electron—to reduce another compound. If a compound donates electrons easily, it has a high reducing power. Antioxidants are able to easily donate electrons to molecules in need of an electron, such as free radicals, before they "steal" one from someplace else, thus continuing the disruptive effects of such thefts on the molecules in question.

Every time molecules lose or gain an electron, the molecules are weakened and, ultimately, the whole structure, whether it is an enzyme, a protein, a cell membrane, tissues, or organ, is damaged. Some areas of the body are more susceptible to damage than others. For example, individuals exposed to high amounts of sunshine are susceptible to skin cancer and cataracts, others who smoke are at risk for lung or throat cancer, others who consume excess alcohol are at risk for liver disease, others still who consume excess protein and fats are subject to elevated homocysteine levels, elevated cholesterol levels and heart disease. Our genetics also plays an important role, as do several hundred other environmental and lifestyle factors.

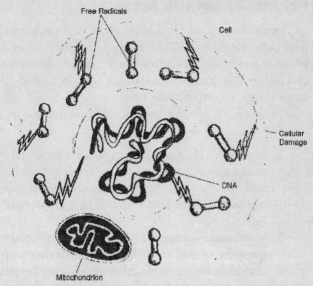

Figure 2—Free Radical Cell Damage.
Free radicals are generated inside the mitochondrion as a part of normal metabolism. The unstable molecules ricochet around the cells, damaging DNA and other structures.

Cell membrane damage can lead to numerous degenerative problems and accelerated aging. Free radicals are major factors in over 80 different diseases and health problems, including heart disease, cancer, diabetes, cataracts, macular degeneration, Alzheimer's, varicose veins, capillary fragility, and inflammatory-related diseases, such as arthritis, lupus, asthma, allergies, and so on.

Free Radicals Accelerate Aging

Aging also results from the loss of vital cells from free radical reactions. With each cell destroyed and without the ability to renew itself, we become one cell older. Free radicals can attack and damage cells from inside or outside the cell.

Free radicals age the body in at least five ways:

1. **Lipid peroxidation.** Free radicals damage fatty compounds (triglycerides or cholesterol) circulating in the bloodstream, causing the release of more free radicals in a chain reaction.

2. **Membrane damage.** Free radicals destroy the integrity of cell membranes, interfering with the cell's ability to absorb nutrients and expel waste products. Without this ability, the cell dies.

3. **Cross-linking.** When free radicals damage molecules in any one cell, other cells split off to repair the injury. As these cells then rejoin with others to reform and reshape themselves, cross linkages may occur. A cross linkage is a bond between large amino acid molecules which are normally separate from each other. Additional free radicals are also formed when waste fragments of these molecules break off. Most people are familiar with cross linkages as a cause of wrinkles, but they also cause "aging" throughout the entire body. Free radicals cause proteins (i.e., collagen tissue) and/or genetic material (i.e., DNA) to fuse. Healthy DNA is necessary to replicate and

renew the body's cellular components. Altered DNA produces useless debris and sometimes cancerous cells.

4. **Lysosomal damage.** Free radicals destroy the membranes of lysosomes, the enzyme-containing organelles found inside most cells. If the membrane sac that stores these enzymes is ruptured, the enzymes will kill the cell.

5. **Miscellaneous reactions.** Miscellaneous free radical reactions form residues called lipofuscin or age pigment. These residues accumulate with time and interfere with cell function and life processes.

Oxygen Free Radicals

We refer to one type of free radical in the body, the toxic oxygen molecules, as oxidants. Many oxidants are actually formed in the body naturally. While we think of oxygen as vital to life, it is also responsible for the destruction and aging of all living things. Similar to the effect where iron is oxidized to rust, oxygen in its toxic state is able to oxidize molecules in our bodies. Compounds which prevent this process are called *antioxidants.*

Production of oxygen-free radicals is a normal part of the body's mechanism. There are tens of thousands of free radicals formed in the body every second. Not all oxygen-free radicals are harmful; some actually help us. The body's immune system uses free radicals to kill potentially infectious microbes and viruses. This activity is known as phagocytosis. At the same time, however, phagocytosis creates even more free radicals (hydrogen peroxide and hydroxyl radicals) that may lead to severe tissue damage.

As long as the ratio of oxidants to antioxidants remains in balance, the negative effects of the free radicals can be controlled. When the balance becomes upset by excessive exposure to internal or external factors or a combination of both, the antioxidants produced by the body simply cannot cope with the increased amount of free radicals. Internal factors here include chronic elevated glucose (as in diabetes) or chronic inflammation. External factors include our daily exposure to environmental free radicals—a major contributor to production of free radicals in the body.

Oxygen-free radicals are formed by molecular oxygen which is reduced in the body to water. The intermediate products formed during oxygen reduction are even more dangerous, including superoxide radicals, hydrogen peroxide, or the extremely damaging hydroxyl radical which reacts with anything it touches. Approximately 5 to 10% of the oxygen we breathe is converted to such radicals.

We are composed of molecules which make up proteins, membranes (consisting of readily oxidizable phospholipids), and polymers (made up of carbohydrates and nucleic acids). These and all other compounds and tissues in the body are susceptible to attack from reactive oxygen radicals.

Different Types of Free Radicals (Oxidants)

There are six different types of free radicals (oxidants):

O_2—*Superoxide radicals.* We continuously form these as a part of cellular energy production and immune response, but they also come from irradiation, car exhaust, cigarette smoke, and ozone. O_2 can be converted by iron or copper to the more toxic OH.

OH—*Hydroxl radicals*—and O_2H_2—*Hydroperoxy radicals* (also known as hydrogen peroxide). These are the most aggressive and damaging species known. These are formed in the body as part of normal metabolism and are particularly harmful to cellular membranes.

NO—*Nitrous oxide.* Reacts with oxygen to form the more damaging oxidant, nitrogen dioxide (NO_2).

NO_2—*Nitrogen dioxide.* Is formed in the body when NO reacts with oxygen. Nitrogen dioxide is a more damaging oxidant compared to NO. Nitrogen dioxide is also a component of pollution, particularly in urban areas. Nitrogen dioxide is particularly stressful to individuals with lung problems. It is found in the body in high levels among asthmatics.

O_3—*Ozone.* An air pollutant which damages the lungs and other tissues.

O—*Singlet oxygen.* Like superoxide radicals, singlet oxygen is produced in the body through various means.

The Antioxidant Players

Antioxidants are a class of nutrients which can destroy free radicals and thus prevent the diseases associated with free radical damage. Antioxidant nutrients also help alleviate the symptoms and side effects of many of these diseases. The following are the major antioxidants of the body:

Vitamin C (ascorbic acid) is effective against hydroxyl and superoxide radicals. Vitamin C also indirectly fights oxidation in the fatty layers of the cells as it converts oxidized vitamin E back to its oxidant form. Humans cannot manufacture vitamin C so it must be provided daily through dietary sources.

Vitamin C is found in many fruits and vegetables including guava, mango, kiwi, oranges, strawberries, broccoli, cauliflower, and brussels sprouts. It is also available as a supplement.

Vitamin E (alpha-tocopherol) is a major fat-soluble antioxidant found within the membranes of cells. It protects the fatty acids, including those in the blood, from damage from peroxyl radicals. Vitamin E is our principal antioxidant against ozone. Vitamin E must be provided daily through dietary sources.

Vitamin E is found in cold-pressed oils from corn, sunflower, safflower, wheat germ, etc., and also eggs, organ meats, molasses, and leafy vegetables.

Beta-carotene, which is just one of about 50 different carotenoids, is effective against singlet oxygen. It is a "weak" antioxidant compared to vitamins E and C. Beta-carotene is one of the few carotenoids which can convert to vitamin A, a fat-soluble antioxidant. Vitamin A is ineffective against singlet oxygen.

Beta-carotene is found in yellow and green fruits

and leafy vegetables such as mango, papaya, cantaloupe, beet greens, spinach, and broccoli. It is also available as a supplement.

Glutathione is composed of three amino acids, cysteine, glutamic acid, and glycine. Glutathione is qualified to act against free radicals which cause the formation of cross-links in collagen tissue. This activity is conducted extracellularly by glutathione against free radical activity as well as lipid peroxidases, which are deactivated. Intracellularly, the activity of a glutathione-related enzyme, **Glutathione peroxidase,** accomplishes the same task. This enzyme is formed by combining glutathione with selenium. Other cofactors include zinc, manganese, and copper. Glutathione also converts oxidized vitamin C back to its oxidant form.

Cysteine, glutamic acid, and glycine are found in protein foods such as milk and other dairy products, meats, and most nuts. Glutathione is available as a dietary supplement.

Methionine has shown protective antioxidant effects against alcohol and also aids in the maintenance of the pool of glutathione peroxidase. Humans cannot manufacture methionine so it must be provided daily through dietary sources including milk and other dairy products, meats, and most nuts. L-methionine is also available as a dietary supplement.

Cysteine is a large part of the enzyme glutathione peroxidase. As an antioxidant detoxification agent, cysteine/cystine has been shown to protect the body against damage induced by alcohol and cigarette smoking, and helps prevent liver and brain damage.

Cystine, which converts to cysteine, is available from protein foods including milk and other dairy products, meats, and most nuts. N-acetyl-cysteine (NAC) is also readily available as a supplement.

Coenzyme Q-10 (Co-Q-10) is an antioxidant that provides protection from oxidative damage occurring in fat-soluble membranes such as cell membranes. Some prescription drugs such as Lovastatin® (commonly prescribed to lower elevated cholesterol), and several psychotropic drugs, including antidepressants, inhibit the manufacture of Co-Q-10 in the body. Supplementation of Co-Q-10 can help prevent some of the side effects of these drugs.

The most abundant food sources of Co-Q-10 are red meat and organ meats.

Alpha Lipoic Acid is both water- and fat-soluble, so is able to protect inside and outside of cells. It is capable of recycling several other antioxidants. Lipoic acid converts into dihydrolipoic acid (DHLA) another antioxidant, which has additional protective benefits.

Alpha Lipoic Acid is found in small amounts in meat, potatoes, carrots, spinach, and many other foods, but to obtain its therapeutic antioxidant effects, one needs to supplement.

Selenium is the principal mineral antioxidant. It is a cofactor in glutathione peroxidase, the body's own free radical controller. Selenium also potentiates the effectiveness of vitamin E against free radicals.

Antioxidant and Enzyme Cellular Protection

Inside and outside cellular membranes

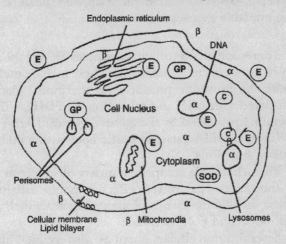

Figure 3—Antioxidant and Enzyme Cellular Protection.
This figure illustrates how the various antioxidants protect
different cellular components.

Selenium is found in tuna, wheat germ, wheat
bran, sesame seeds, pecans, Brazil nuts, and meats.
It is also available as a supplement.

Zinc serves as an antioxidant by stimulating the
activity of **superoxide dismutase (SOD),** which is considered the second most important antioxidant produced by the body, following glutathione.

Zinc is found in pumkin seeds, sunflower seeds, seafood, organ meats, mushrooms, brewer's yeast, soybeans, oysters, eggs, wheat germ, and meats. It is also available as a supplement.

There are many other substances in the body which also serve as antioxidants. These include **melatonin,** the hormone produced by the pineal gland associated with sleep and relaxation, and DHEA, the hormone produced by the adrenal glands. DHEA is the most abundant steriod in the body with a multitude of functions.

Phytochemicals comprise a variety of supplemental substances that are very effective as antioxidants. These include thousands of plant chemicals such as flavonoids and polyphenolics.

Several intracellular enzymes also reduce the harmful effects of free radicals of oxidants inside the cell. These are **glutathione peroxidase** (found in the mitochondria and cytosol), **catalase** (found in peroxisomes and breaks down hydrogen to oxygen and water), and **SOD** (present in cytosol, a copper/zinc dependent enzyme) and mitochondria (a manganese-dependent enzyme).

The following increase your need for antioxidants:

1. Exercise.
2. Stress.
3. Exposure to pollutants, smog, poisons; e.g., tobacco, smoke, alcohol, drugs, and pesticides.
4. Illness, infection, inflammation, and many

health problems: e.g., diabetes, arthritis, and asthma.

5. Elevated blood lipids (especially LDL) and elevated blood sugar.
6. Many stimulants and metabolic enhancers such as caffeine and diet pills.
7. Radiation (including UV light from the sun).

Some scientists believe that the reason humans live longer than chimpanzees, cats, dogs and other mammals is that we have a higher level of antioxidants within our cells (Culter). Perhaps people who live longer than others is also because they have higher levels of antioxidants within their cells protecting them from damage and disease.

Your Antioxidant Profile

Your antioxidant profile can tell a great deal about how well you are protecting your overall health by protecting the health of your cells. To learn where you stand, take the following quiz.

Answer each of the following questions by circling the correct response for you. Then calculate your score by checking your answers at the end of this quiz.

1. How many servings of yellow-orange fruits and leafy green or yellow-orange vegetables do you have daily?
a. 2 to 4 half-cup or equivalent size servings
b. 5 to 9 half-cup or equivalent size servings
c. less than 2 half-cup servings

2. *Are the vegetables that you eat mostly fried, baked, boiled, steamed, or raw?*
   a. fried
   b. baked
   c. boiled
   d. steamed
   e. raw

3. *Do you use "cold-pressed" vegetable oil?*
   a. yes
   b. no

4. *How often do you travel by airplane?*
   a. more than 6 times a month
   b. about 2 to 4 times a month
   c. less than once a month

5. *How much time do you spend outdoors?*
   a. more than 20 hours a week
   b. about 5 to 20 hours a week
   c. less than 5 hours a week

6. *Do you smoke cigarettes?*
   a. yes
   b. no

7. *Do you have more than one or two alcoholic beverages a day?*
   a. yes
   b. no

8. *How close do you live to a city or industrial manufacturing complex?*

a. live in city or near an industrial manufacturing complex
b. live in suburbs of city or several miles away from an industrial manufacturing complex
c. live in rural area, far from a city or an industrial manufacturing complex

9. How often do you exercise?

a. more than 5 times a week, each session lasting more than 30 minutes
b. 3 or 4 times a week, for about 30 minutes per session
c. less than 2 times a week

10. Are you taking an antioxidant formula to supplement your diet?

a. yes
b. no

YOUR SCORE

Each response is given a numeric value. A value of 5 is the most positive, and lower values may indicate areas that need improvement. After answering the questions, add up the score as given to determine your Antioxidant Profile.

Question 1.

a. 2   You are not obtaining protective amounts of antioxidants from fruits and vegetables, leaving cells vulnerable to free radical destruction; eat three to five more servings a day.
b. 5   You're getting valuable antioxidants from fruits and vegetables, especially if the vegetables are eaten raw.

c. 0 You're not getting any antioxidants from fruits and vegetables; to help protect cells from free radical damage, eat five to nine servings a day.

Question 2.
a. 1 Frying is high in fat; heat destroys some antioxidants.
b. 3 Baking is healthy, but usually requires the addition of fat, and involves the loss of some antioxidants to heat.
c. 2 Antioxidants are lost through leaching and heat.
d. 4 Steaming is a healthy cooking option, but it destroys some antioxidants.
e. 5 Raw, fresh vegetables supply the most intact antioxidants.

Question 3.
a. 5 More vitamin E remains in cold-pressed vegetable oil than in oil processed with heat.
b. 0 Certain vegetable oils are good sources of polyunsaturated fats, which are associated with helping to lower cholesterol levels. However, heat processing destroys vitamin E, increasing your need for this vitamin.

Question 4.
a. 0 Research indicates that airline passengers may be exposed to relatively high levels of radiation; the more one flies, the greater the exposure. Studies show that radiation may be associated with increased free radical activity,

increasing the need for cell-protecting antioxidants.

b. 3   Moderate air travel exposes passengers to greater levels of radiation than if traveling by ground transportation. Even this amount of radiation exposure affects free radical activity, increasing the need for antioxidants.

c. 5   Limited air travel lessens your exposure to elevated radiation levels associated with airline flights; therefore, your requirement for antioxidants is not affected by this activity.

Question 5.

a. 1   Excessive exposure to sunlight and ambient radiation may increase free radical activity, possibly increasing the need for protective antioxidants.

b. 2   Moderate exposure to sunlight and ambient radiation may have an effect on free radical activity, possibly increasing the need for protective antioxidants.

c. 5   Limited outdoor activity decreases your exposure to the harmful effects of the sun.

Question 6.

a. 0   Smoking may greatly increase the need for protective antioxidants. Vitamins E and C work synergistically to protect lung cells from free radical activity caused by smoking.

b. 5   Yet another good reason not to smoke, as research shows that it may increase the need for antioxidants.

Question 7.

   a. 0 High intakes of alcohol may greatly increase the need for all the antioxidants, particularly selenium. Moreover, all nutrients may be affected by high alcohol intake.

   b. 5 Moderate to no intake of alcohol does not affect your requirement for antioxidants.

Question 8.

   a. 2 Air pollution may increase your need for antioxidants.

   b. 3 You may be exposed to some of the air pollution from a nearby city or industrial manufacturing plant.

   c. 5 Even when living in a pollution-free environment, normal body metabolism requires antioxidants to battle free radicals.

Question 9.

   a. 3 Excessive exercise increases your need for many nutrients, including antioxidants.

   b. 4 Although exercise increases your need for antioxidants, experts recommend a moderate exercise program to maintain good health. Adding a vitamin and mineral supplement ensures protective amounts of antioxidants, particularly during physical stress.

   c. 5 Exercise increases the need for antioxidants. By not exercising regularly, however, you are likely to have more body fat, be overweight, and have an increased risk of associated diseases.

Question 10.
  a. 5 You are assured of getting the protective amounts of antioxidants.
  b. 0 You may not be getting protective amounts of antioxidants every day.

Your Antioxidant Profile

45 to 50: Excellent. You know how to live a healthy lifestyle and protect your cells with a diet rich in antioxidants—the nutrients that research shows may help to protect your body's cells from the ravaging effects of free radicals.

35 to 45: You are on the right track, but you may need to strengthen your cell-protecting antioxidant profile. Review the questions, and determine which areas need greater attention.

Less than 35: You need help. By improving your antioxidant profile, you will help prevent the destructive damage of natural body processes on cells.

CHAPTER 3

Free Radical Diseases

The Mayo Clinic reports that approximately 43% of deaths in the United States are due to some form of cardiovascular disease, and 23% are caused by cancer. This is two of every three deaths.

We now see the critical role which free radicals play in the development of both diseases. Low levels of antioxidants, which increase free radical activity, are clearly associated with an increased risk of these diseases. By using antioxidant supplements to scavenge free radicals, a person can potentially decrease the risks of cancer, cardiovascular disease, and many other degenerative health problems (Barber and Harris).

Although we do not yet fully understand exactly how free radicals cause oxidative damage to cells and tissues, we know that they do so. In general, these radicals act on different structures, and the use of various antioxidants exerts favorable countereffects. Our genetics may make us sensitive to certain health problems such as heart disease or diabetes, but the location of exposure to or origin of free radicals also plays a significant role in the type of damage which results. For example, UV exposure is damaging to the skin and the eyes, and elevated LDL cholesterol molecules circulating in our veins are more susceptible to forming arterial plaque. Smoking, of course, damages the throat and lungs, and so on.

Free Radicals Attack Three Types of Molecules

1. **Polyunsaturated fatty acids:** Free radicals destroy cell membranes which are made up of these sensitive fatty acids. Free radicals also damage LDL and lipoprotein(a), which are associated with heart disease.
2. **DNA:** Damage to genetic material is associated with cell death, cell abnormalities, and cancer.
3. **Proteins:** Protein destruction is seen in cataract formation, kidney damage, and damage to hemoglobin cells and aging in general (collagen breakdown).
(See diagram, p. 38.)

Are You a Victim of Free Radical Attack?

Do you bruise easily?

Capillary fragility is the result of free radical damage upon the capillaries. Fragile capillaries are prone to leak blood with the slightest bump. If you do have many bruises, you may not even remember how you obtained them because the bump seemed insignificant at the time.

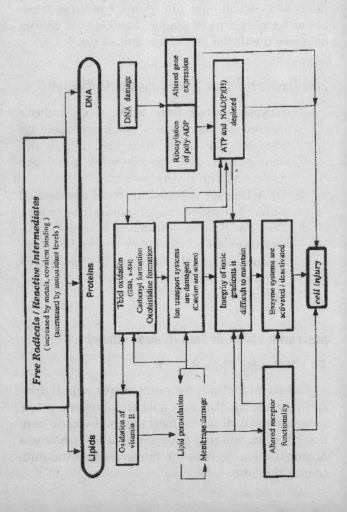

Do you have a lot of wrinkles?

When collagen tissues breakdown in the skin, you will have wrinkles. UV radiation causes free radical formation at the skin and rapid depletion of antioxidant supplies in these areas as well.

Do you have heart disease?

Oxidation of low-density lipoproteins (LDL) (the "bad" cholesterol) creates free radicals and a chain reaction of events resulting in plaque buildup and clogged arteries.

Do you have arthritis?

The pain and swelling of arthritis is also caused by free radicals, which generate more free radicals and the release of harmful inflammatory prostaglandins in tissues.

Do you have cancer?

There are probably over 100 different types of cancer and probably hundreds of ways which free radicals can cause damage associated with cancer. Here are just a few examples.

Carcinogens and many other things such as radiation (including sunlight) form free radicals in the body and can activate oncogenes which cause cancer.

Free radicals can also damage sensors on cell membranes that regulate cell growth and proliferation. If sensors are damaged, unregulated growth can occur. Unregulated growth and cancer go hand in hand.

Free radicals can damage the genetic material (DNA in the nucleus), causing mutation of the cell.

Free radicals can also damage components of the immune system such as white blood cells or enzymes which would otherwise recognize and destroy mutated cells before they multiply and become cancerous.

Do you have cataracts?

The sensitive protein and fatty acid tissues in the eye are highly susceptible to free radical damage if there are inadequate levels of antioxidants to stop the damage. Excess sunlight is a risk factor for cataracts. Free radicals created by sunlight and other factors can also damage the retina, causing retinopathy, or the macula, causing macular degeneration.

Do you have HIV?

Studies show that individuals with human immunodeficiency virus (HIV) have lower levels of various antioxidants compared to individuals without HIV. This further compromises one's state of health and susceptibility to illness.

Do you have allergies or asthma?

Epidemiological studies show associations among oxidant exposure, respiratory infections, and asthma in children of smokers. Symptoms of ongoing asthma in adults appear to be increased by exposure to environmental oxidants and decreased by antioxidant supplementation. There is evidence that oxidants produced in the body by overactive inflammatory cells contribute to ongoing asthma and allergic hypersensitivities (Hatch).

Do you have a sprain or other injury— laceration, etc.?

Anytime there is tissue damage due to a cut or fall, the surrounding area tissues generate more free radicals through the release of inflammatory hormone-like substances called prostaglandins.

Are you experiencing memory loss, Alzheimer's, etc.?

While it is not known entirely what the exact causes of Alzheimer's, memory loss, and senile dementia are, it is known that free radical damage is responsible for neuron degeneration (Behl).

Are you aging "prematurely"?

Cellular damage by oxygen radicals is believed to be directly involved in aging, causing the pathological changes associated with aging. The higher the level of free radicals we have in our cells, the faster we age (Packer).

As we age, we become more susceptible to "age-related diseases" such as diabetes, arthritis, vascular diseases (including coronary artery disease), and hypertension. Interestingly enough, we know now that with antioxidants, these are all, to some extent, preventable!

While the simple life-necessitating acts of breathing and eating create free radicals in the body, many

environmental factors and exposure to various substances increases our exposure to these reactive
chemical structures. Some of these include:

Cigarette smoke
Rancid foods
Rancid fats—trans fatty acids found in margarine,
    and other hydrogenated fats, etc.
Poor diet—especially a diet high in sugar
Certain prescription drugs
Metabolic stimulants such as caffeine, cocaine, nic-
    otine, etc.
Alcohol
Car exhaust
Smog
Air pollutants
Pesticides/herbicides
Ultraviolet light
X rays
Gamma radiation
Strenuous exercise
Stress

How Free Radicals Work

The reaction of oxygen upon molecules in the
body is as essential for aerobic life as it is involved
in numerous other vital processes, such as normal
metabolism. These reactions give rise to a variety of
reactive oxygen species (ROS), simply identified as
free radicals. Keeping these activating reactions (the
creation of free radicals) under control through
detoxification reactions and protective systems is of

great importance. A lack of protective or repair capacity results in cell and tissue damage.

Free Radicals Impair Our Immune System

Now the health or integrity of the membrane determines the cell's ability to function properly. For example, the phagocyte (or activated white blood cell) can move toward an invading bacterium only when its cell membrane is intact. Communication between cells in tissues and the cell's ability to recognize and identify other cells also depends on the health of the cellular membrane. Our immune system itself, which works by seeking out and destroying invaders, can be greatly affected by overinteraction with free radicals. If the free radicals cannot be identified as harmful, they will not be destroyed but will multiply, causing all sorts of problems.

Some cells, such as a heart muscle cell or a liver cell, may become irreversibly damaged when exposed to oxidative stress. After the membrane structure is disrupted, the cell is no longer able to accomplish its functions. If the damaged cells then are not removed by phagocytes, the result may even be malignant transformation of the cell, a possible precursor to cancer.

Certainly the damage free radicals produce varies depending on the site of the attack. As free radicals damage membranes (creating capillary fragility associated with cardiovascular disease), they also can damage ocular lens proteins (creating cataracts), and break down elastin and collagen (associated with aging and wrinkles).

With regard to inflammatory, immunoreactive

damage, radicals are produced by activated white blood cells (phagocytes). When tissue inflammation becomes chronic, for example, oxygen turnover is increased a hundredfold and tissues are flooded with free radicals.

Free Radicals Destroy Proteins/DNA

In addition to damaging membranes, free radicals may also destroy proteins, which can then lead to specific diseases depending on the type of protein. When proteins are affected, metabolic disorders can develop. When DNA is affected and lesions appear within the DNA, increased rates of metagenesis and carcinogenesis can develop. Thus, a broad spectrum of injuries may occur in tissues as a result of enhanced radical formation.

Remember this, though: direct radical attack to the DNA can result in an increase in *cancer incidence*. There is sufficient evidence for a relation between free radicals and cancer at least from in vitro experiments, animal studies, and epidemiologic trials to note this disturbing fact. Cancer is most certainly a "free-radical associated disease."

Free Radicals and Heart Disease

Free radicals also play a role in the development of atherosclerosis by attacking the plasma lipoproteins. After being damaged by free radical attack, the atherogenic low-density lipoprotein (LDL), a form of cholesterol, can no longer be recognized by LDL receptors. Considered as a foreign substance, it is then attacked by phagocytes. For their part foam cells are the first sign of an atherosclerotic lesion, representing macrophages which have incorporated oxidized LDL and, through migration into the vessel wall and production of growth factors, produce an early lesion that develops into an atherosclerotic plaque.

Homocysteine is another by-product of protein metabolism which binds with LDL cholesterol causing oxidative damage to the arterial wall, leading to plaque buildup and atherosclerosis. High levels of homocysteine largely result from dietary inadequacies of B_6, B_{12}, folic acid, and trimethylglycine, also known as TMG or betaine.

Homocysteine thiolactone is a highly reactive form of homocysteine which, when released into the bloodstream, causes LDL cholesterol to aggregate. These aggregates are taken up by macrophages (white blood cells) of the artery wall which then form foam cells. Foam cells break down the aggregates and release fats and cholesterol into developing plaques. Foam cells also release homocysteine thiolactone into the surrounding cells, creating free radicals which damage the lining cells or the artery wall. This is the beginning of arteriosclerosis and increased risk for blood clot formation, among other effects.

Studies show that all men (compared to women) and older individuals (both men and women) tend to have higher levels of homocysteine. Studies also show that the higher the level of homocysteine, the higher the risk of heart problems. The higher your level of folic acid, the lower the level of homocysteine. Therefore, increasing your levels of folic acid can prevent a buildup of homocysteine in the blood. Individuals with a high-protein diet also have an increased need for nutrients to help lower elevated homocysteine: vitamin B_6, B_{12}, folic acid, and trimethylglycine (also known as betaine). Antioxidants help reduce free radical damage.

Free Radicals and Arthritis

The cause and progression of the degenerative processes within joint cavities as in arthritis and osteoarthritis are due, at least in part, to the destructive activity of oxygen radicals (Elstner). Studies (in vivo) show that the breakdown of hyaluronic acid by oxygen radicals (OH-) appears to play a role in the loss of function of synovial fluid, a joint lubricant (Peroxinorm). Without this protective fluid to cushion the joints, pain, inflammation, and scar tissue develop.

To make things worse, more free radicals are produced by activated phagocytes due to the inflammation. Oxygen turnover is increased in these situations and tissues are literally flooded with free radicals, creating an endless destructive cycle. Thus we have covered the term "degenerative" to describe conditions that progressively worsen.

Free Radicals and Neurological Damage

Nerve tissue is especially susceptible to radical attack because of its high phospholipid content. Additionally, because of the high energy turnover in the brain (cerebrum) and the extensive oxygen supply required, this tissue is also particularly susceptible to damage. Higher energy requires higher levels of antioxidants to balance the higher level of oxidants produced.

In this regard, a number of disease conditions

are associated with low levels of antioxidants, which creates an increased risk for degenerative nerve conditions. Due to the growing number of "seniors" in our population, the neurodegenerative disorders, such as senile dementia, Parkinson's disease, and Alzheimer's disease, are a very important group of diseases with increasing significance.

But why these diseases develop in the brain can also be related to the presence of specific heavy metals there and the fact that they may activate oxygen. We now know that certain transition metals are greatly concentrated in some regions of the brain, and that is why damage to these regions develops so quickly.

Free Radicals and Sugar

High blood sugar levels can cause protein damage via the creation of destructive oxygen radicals. The nonenzymatic joining of sugar to protein forms these radicals. The process of forming sugar-damaged proteins is called *glycation,* which can be compared to how sliced apples react to air: they brown up and do so very quickly.

Blood sugar (glucose) and some other sugars react spontaneously with collagen, a major protein found in skin, blood vessels and connective tissue, and other proteins to form cross-linked sugar-damaged proteins. These are called *advanced glycosylation end products* (AGEs). When AGEs are formed, additional free radicals are released as well (Tritschler).

The formation rate of AGEs (and free radicals) increases as the blood sugar level increases and the length of time the level is raised increases.

Blood Sugar, Aging, and Disease

Elevated sugar levels are very damaging to the protein tissues in the body. The spontaneous reaction of sugar with tissue proteins such as collagen and myelin is responsible for accelerated tissue aging in diabetics. It is also believed responsible for kidney damage, and is involved in the atherosclerosis process, both common complications of diabetes. In addition, glycation reactions play a role in the normal aging of tissue. Recent studies show that diabetics as well as aging animals do indeed have increased concentrations of AGEs in their collagen.

As we age, our average blood sugar level tends to rise. This is because our tissues become less sensitive to the actions of insulin as we get older. Such desensitization creates higher levels of free radicals and a greater need for antioxidant supplementation.

The roles that oxygen and sugar-damaged protein play with regard to protein tissues does explain much of the secondary aging effects and some of the primary aging process. Maintaining even and optimal blood sugar levels (70 to 100 mg per dl.), as well as adequate antioxidant protection throughout life, can protect our tissues from "aging" prematurely.

Antioxidants and Antiglycation

Both free radical reduction and glycation reduction (through antioxidants) reduce the incidence of the aging diseases, including heart disease, arthritis, and cancer. They are complementary approaches that enhance each other's benefits. It is important to note as well that antioxidant protection against free radical damage is more efficient with both approaches than through the actions of either alone.

Of course, some cellular damage caused by radicals can be repaired by enzymes. We actually produce some of these enzymes in the body for the sole purpose of repairing damage to cells caused by radicals and by high levels of blood sugar. Nonetheless, it is still necessary to sustain adequate levels of antioxidants to protect these organic enzymes from free radical damage.

Cellular Protection Systems

As just noted, our cells do not lack protection against free radicals. Protection and repair systems are available which, within their capacity limits, allow oxygen activation to occur with no resulting damage. Among these protection systems are enzymes like superoxide dismutase (SOD), catalase, peroxidases, and glutathione peroxidase. In addition, in plants as well as in animals, there are metabolites such as ascorbic acid (vitamin C), alpha-tocopherol (vitamin E), sulphur-containing amino acids like cysteine and glutathione, and various carotenoids, odiphenoles and sugars which act as radical scavengers.

The goal is to obtain a balance between oxidants and antioxidants in the body. If you have more oxidants than you do antioxidants, the result is damage to your cells and tissues. On the other hand, if the level of antioxidants in the body is higher than the level of free radicals, the excess antioxidants may actually create free radicals.

CHAPTER 4

The Perfect Antioxidant: Alpha Lipoic Acid

Supplemental antioxidants are useful to keep free radicals in check and to maintain good health. Although there is no one single, perfect antioxidant, Alpha Lipoic Acid is a candidate which approaches that ideal. Understand though that antioxidant nutrients are partners working together. Vitamins C, E, and A are essential vitamins as well as antioxidants. They all work better, however, when Alpha Lipoic Acid is available in levels where it can be used as an antioxidant, not merely tied up as a coenzyme that helps to facilitate the work of the metabolism.

Dr. Lester Packer, Professor at the University of California, Berkeley, Department of Molecular and Cell Biology, among the world's leading antioxidant researchers, is also perhaps the foremost researcher on Alpha Lipoic Acid. He has described an ideal antioxidant as one that has the following biochemical properties:

1. Quenches a variety of oxidative species.
2. Is easily absorbed and is readily bioavailable.
3. Exists in a variety of locations: tissues, cells, extracellular fluid, intracellular fluid, various membranes, etc.
4. Interacts with other antioxidants.
5. Chelates free metal ions.
6. Has positive effects on gene expression.

Alpha Lipoic Acid and DHLA (the reduced form of Alpha Lipoic Acid) do all of the above very well.

Alpha Lipoic Acid: The Ultimate Antioxidant

Alpha Lipoic Acid is the ideal antioxidant because it is both water- and fat-soluble, works inside and outside of cells, participates in redox cycling by breaking down to Dihydrolipoic Acid (DHLA) which recharges other important antioxidants, and quenches several different types of free radicals. Taken together, this combined effect works well to combat almost all species of free radicals.

Alpha Lipoic Acid terminates the hydroxyl and hypochlorous free radicals. Its reduced form, DHLA, terminates hydroxyl and hypochlorous free radicals and, in addition, terminates superoxide free radicals and peroxyl free radicals. Alpha Lipoic Acid also quenches the reactive oxygen species singlet oxygen and possibly hydrogen peroxide in some domains but not in others.

In addition, Alpha Lipoic Acid can partially replace some of the dietary need for vitamins C and E. In 1959, Drs. Rosenberg and Culik showed that

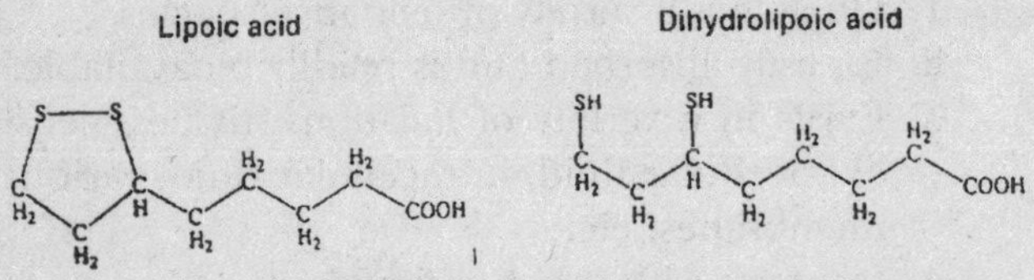

Lipoic acid   Dihydrolipoic acid

Figure 5—Thiotic Acid (Lipoic Acid) Molecular Configuration.
The structures of alpha lipoic acid and dihydrolipoic acid,
shown as chemical structures.

Alpha Lipoic Acid prevented scurvy in vitamin C–
deficient animals and that it prevented symptoms
of vitamin E deficiency in laboratory animals fed a
vitamin E–deficient diet. They even predicted that
Alpha Lipoic Acid might act as an antioxidant for
vitamins C and E.

What Makes Alpha Lipoic Acid So Special?

1. The structure of Alpha Lipoic Acid is very small,
which allows it to easily slip through cell membranes,
providing antioxidant protection on both the inside
and outside of cells. Many other antioxidants are too
large to pass through the cell membrane and thus
offer protection only on the outside of the cell.

2. Alpha Lipoic Acid possesses antioxidant prop-
erties in its original form and *also* in its reduced form,
DHLA. Alpha Lipoic Acid is readily converted to
DHLA after being ingested as a supplement.

Most antioxidant substances can act as antioxidants only in their reduced forms. After they have
donated an electron, they are then "used up" unless
they are regenerated by another antioxidant (like
Alpha Lipoic Acid).

As you can see from this table, many different types of free radicals can be prevented from causing damage through Alpha Lipoic Acid either on its own or through its conversion in the body to DHLA.

Name of Free Radical	Terminated by Alpha Lipoic Acid through donation of electron	Terminated by DHLA through donation of electron
Superoxide (O_2)	No	?
Hydroxy radical (HO)	Yes	Yes
Peroxyl radical (ROO)	Possibly	Possibly
Hypochlorous radical (HOCL)	Yes	Yes
Singlet oxygen	Yes	Yes
Hydrogen peroxide (H_2O_2)	No	No
Heavy metals (Fe, Cu, Cd, Pb, Hg)	Chelated*	Chelated*

*Chelation refers to the ability to "chelate" or grab hold of metallic substances that might otherwise cause toxicity, contribute to plaque formation, or oxidize and create more free radicals.

3. In its oxidized form, surface atoms at the end of the molecule form a ring structure known as the dithiole ring. (A disulfide molecule located in this ring allows Alpha Lipoic Acid to act as an enzyme catalyst.) When this ring is broken, either through oxidation or through enzymes, the result is Dihydrolipoic Acid (DHLA), which is an even more potent antioxidant than Alpha Lipoic Acid.

4. Alpha Lipoic Acid functions in the body as an antioxidant and in other ways. First, Alpha Lipoic

Acid is a coenzyme in the metabolic process; specifically it is necessary for the conversion of glucose to energy (ATP). Small amounts of Alpha Lipoic Acid are bound chemically at the active sites of enzymes. Second, when taken as a supplement and higher levels of concentration build up in the body, Alpha Lipoic Acid can act as a potent antioxidant itself.

Alpha Lipoic Acid Recycles

When an antioxidant such as vitamin E donates an electron to a radical, the vitamin E is oxidized and the radical is reduced. If the vitamin E does not receive another electron from another molecule, it is used up. If the vitamin E is reduced, it recycles back to its original form.

Lipoic Acid has a very low redox potential. This means that in its reduced form (DHLA), it very readily donates electrons to either stabilize a radical or recycle an oxidized molecule (like vitamin C). Thus, Alpha Lipoic Acid can not only terminate free radicals, but can also regenerate other antioxidants in the body and allow them to scavenge free radicals at will.

As we know, the body is most inventive in combatting disease and breakdown. It is in its very nature to do so. For example, the body produces enzymes (superoxide dismutase, glutathione peroxidase, and catalase) which protect us from free radical damage. But we can also help the body and protect ourselves through eating foods with high amounts of antioxidants or by taking supplemental nutrients such as ascorbic acid, α-tocopherol, or the carotenoids. The body also requires other nutrients to help it either manufacture these substances or to utilize them. These include zinc, copper, manganese in the case of superoxide dismutase, or selenium and cysteine in the case of glutathione peroxidase.

Significance of Glutathione

Glutathione peroxidase (composed of the amino acids glutamic acid, cysteine, and glycine) is the premier antioxidant enzyme in the body. It plays an important role in cell detoxification, heavy metal detoxification, immune function, DNA and protein synthesis, transport processes, and the removal of free radicals.

Glutathione peroxidase not only eliminates hydrogen peroxide but also repairs damage which has already occurred. Following the oxidation of fatty acids to hydroperoxides, glutathione peroxidase prevents this activity from continuing any further. It is a true repair enzyme for membrane lesions. Ascorbic acid, alpha-tocopherol, and the carotenoids can reduce free radicals directly by sacrificing an electron.

Glutathione levels tend to drop as we get older, about 3–4% every decade from age 20 to 70. While this lifelong decrease may not seem important, we know in fact that it is. Low levels of glutathione levels are associated with numerous health problems, including diabetes, cardiovascular disease, arthritis, cataracts, and increased susceptibility to health problems in general.

Research shows that low glutathione levels were

one of the three variables in elderly people to demonstrate a negative effect on susceptibility to illness and survival. The other two variables were age and suppressed anger. Higher glutathione levels were associated with a lower number of illnesses, higher levels of self-rated health, lower cholesterol, lower body mass index, and lower blood pressure (Julius et al., Lang et al.).

Glutathione synthesis in the body is dependent upon the intracellular availability of cysteine, an essential amino acid. Lester Packer has reported that administration of Alpha Lipoic Acid is beneficial in several oxidative stress situations probably because of an increase in cellular glutathione content. Just recently, however, German researchers demonstrated that this increase is due to an enhanced cysteine supply following administration of DHLA (Kis et al.).

In brief, then, glutathione and the relationship between glutathione and cysteine are significant for these reasons:

- Glutathione in both its oxidized and reduced form functions very similarly to the manner in which Alpha Lipoic Acid/DHLA functions.
- Glutamic acid passes the blood brain barrier and is considered "brain fuel." It is necessary for a healthy brain and a healthy attitude, too!
- Glutamic acid gives rise to GABA (a calming agent in the brain) and possibly to neurotransmitters.
- Glutamic acid is a component of folic acid, a member of the B complex family. Folic acid is needed to produce hemoglobin, the oxygen-

transporting cells in the blood; causes the production of hydrochloric acid in the stomach; and helps lower elevated homocysteine levels. Elevated homocysteine levels are associated with increased risk for cardiovascular disease.

- Glutamic acid and also cysteine are necessary for glucose regulation.
- Glutamic acid and cysteine protect against the effects of alcohol and smoking. Glutamic acid can also decrease cravings for alcohol and, sometimes, sugar.
- Cysteine is necessary for production of glutathione in the body.
- Cysteine removes heavy metal deposits.
- Cysteine production in the body is inhibited by chronic illness.

Low Levels of Glutathione and Cysteine Are Associated with Health Problems

Reduced levels of glutathione (as well as a number of other antioxidants) are seen among individuals with many health problems. These include:

Diabetes	*Cardiovascular disease*
HIV	*Chronic fatigue*
Asthma	*Osteoporosis*
Allergies	*Kidney disease*
Arthritis	*Lupus*
Alcoholism	*(Also, chronic crankiness!)*

Alpha Lipoic Acid Increases Glutathione Levels

As part of its regeneration of its partner antioxidant, Alpha Lipoic Acid also increases cellular glutathione content. Glutathione, a major antioxidant within cells, is the major repair enzyme.

Glutathione and Alpha Lipoic Acid Regenerate Vitamin E

As a fat-soluble substance, vitamin E is one of the major protectors of polyunsaturated fatty acids from free radical damage. Membranes, largely composed of polyunsaturated fatty acids, possess many double bonds, and radical chain reactions are easily initiated under the influence of oxygen, leading to an oxidation process that sweeps across the membrane.

To stop the chain reaction, some kinds of "radical extinguishers" (such as vitamin E) are naturally incorporated in the membrane. The radical chain reaction ends at the place on the membrane where a vitamin E molecule is situated.

For example, low-density lipoprotein (LDL), the cholesterol often referred to as the "bad" cholesterol, is highly susceptible to such damage. Each LDL, which consists of about 1,300 molecules, contains almost 7.5 moles of antioxidants (mostly α-tocopherol, a form of vitamin E). As the vitamin E is oxidized, by being used to stop free radicals), its protective activity is lost. The lower the level of vitamin E, the less protection we have against free radical damage. (This is why E is so important to protect us against heart disease.) Regeneration of the E molecule can occur through glutathione peroxidase and ascorbic acid, but as they do so, they too are oxidized and used up.

Obviously, increasing the amount of vitamin E would therefore provide us with increased protection against damage. The good news is that if Alpha Lipoic Acid, glutathione, and vitamin C are present, they synergistically are able to protect us against the loss of vitamin E. They are able to donate an electron so that its protective properties are restored (or recycled). This means that it takes longer for the free radicals to damage the molecule.

As vitamin C and glutathione are not fat-soluable, they do not directly protect areas which require a fat-soluable substance, but they can enhance the action of Vitamin E, which does protect such areas. Remember, Alpha Lipoic Acid is both fat- and water-soluble.

Exposure to an Oxidant ⟶ Loss of E	
If no protection is added:	**100%**
If dihydrolipoate (DHLA) is added:	90%
If ascorbate (vitamin C) is added:	60%
If both vitamin C and dihydrolipoate (DHLA) are added:	**30%**

(Packer, L., *The Vitamin E, Ascorbate and Alpha Lipoic Acid Antioxidant Defense System.*)

Alpha Lipoic Acid/DHLA Work with Vitamins C and E

The direct free radical–scavenging effect of DHLA is not the only mode of its antioxidant action. DHLA can also synergistically enhance the antioxidant protective activity of cell membranes by recycling tocopherol radicals and working synergistically with vitamin C (Bast and Haenen; Scholich).

Dr. Packer reports that the research he has done leaves little doubt about the antioxidant effectiveness of DHLA, which can directly scavenge peroxyl and superoxide radicals and/or enhance other water- or lipid-soluble antioxidants (ascorbate and vitamin E) by regenerating them via the reduction of their radicals.

The Alpha Lipoic Acid/DHLA redox couple has been found to exert a synergistic action in the antioxidant-recycling mechanisms of natural membranes and LDL in vitro and in protecting against oxidative injury.

When antioxidants have a high affinity for certain free radicals, they are recognized as part of the *thiol antioxidant system*. Glutathione is also part of this system as dihydrolipoate has a similar recycling effect on glutathione. Alpha Lipoic Acid is also known as Thioctic Acid.

One can predict that protection should be increased by bolstering antioxidant defenses. Researchers have tested this hypothesis and demonstrated that Alpha Lipoic Acid supplementation protects tissues in organs such as the liver, heart, brain, and skin against lipid peroxidation induced by peroxyl radicals.

Because of the association of disease with the significant damage to membrane phospholipids from free radical peroxidation, researchers are feverishly examining the antioxidant effects of Alpha Lipoic Acid and DHLA (Bast, Scholich, Muller, Bonomi, DeMascio).

Alpha Lipoic Acid Prevents Glycation

Alpha Lipoic Acid effectively reduces the protein damage that high blood sugar levels cause. With Alpha Lipoic Acid's antiglycation action to prevent the damage from blood sugar, and its antioxidant action to protect against free radicals, the minor damage that does occur can be repaired by the still-functioning enzymes in the body. As a result, the cell is protected and the body does not become damaged and thereby one cell older.

DHLA: Fat- and Water-Soluble

Alpha Lipoic Acid alone is not effective in scavenging all types of free radicals. For example, Alpha Lipoic Acid is not effective against peroxyl radicals. In the body, however, Alpha Lipoic Acid readily converts to DHLA which can usually ward off damage by functioning as a scavenger against water-soluble and lipid-soluble radicals. This is the only known antioxidant which has this special property of acting in both water- and fat-soluble mediums.

In contrast to many other antioxidants, DHLA may function as a universal free radical quencher which can scavenge radicals in areas where other antioxidants cannot.

Alpha Lipoic Acid: Therapeutic Uses

Alpha Lipoic Acid is currently used as a therapeutic agent in a variety of diseases, including liver and neurological disorders. Patients diagnosed with liver cirrhosis, diabetes, atherosclerosis, and polyneuritis have been found to contain a reduced level of Alpha Lipoic Acid in the body (Altenkirch et al.; Piering and Bratanow).

Inside the cell, DHLA is even more potent than Alpha Lipoic Acid in performing antioxidant functions. DHLA directly destroys damaging superoxide radicals, hydroperoxy radicals and hydroxyl radicals.

In order to perform this antioxidant function in the body, Alpha Lipoic Acid must be present in amounts significantly higher than normal. For the average well person, then, daily supplementation at 100 to 200 mg is sufficient as a preventable dosage. Although Alpha Lipoic Acid is found in many foods, it would be almost impossible to obtain these amounts through the diet alone.

Certainly therapeutic doses can rise much higher. Some studies use daily dosages as high as 600 to 800 mg to reverse symptoms from neuropathy, to assist diabetics with other complications such as cataracts or macular degeneration, or to assist the body in fighting off HIV. Side effects even at these higher dosages are practically nonexistent. Neither have toxic effects been reported as yet.

CHAPTER 5

Antiaging Effects

Aging can be defined as the accumulation of diverse adverse changes that increase the risk of death. Among the several theories that now account for the aging process is the free-radical theory of aging (Harmon). This theory is based on the chemical nature of free radical reactions and their ubiquitous presence in living things. As these reactions occur continuously, they also arise for the most part from oxygen in the course of normal metabolism. The theory goes on to describe how these reactions are countered by enzymatic (glutathione peroxidase and catalase) and nonenzymatic means (vitamins A, C, E; selenium; zinc; Alpha Lipoic Acid; etc.)

With age, we produce higher levels of free radicals in the body. One way to slow down this production of oxidants is through calorie restriction.

Researchers have shown that reducing caloric intake by one third will substantially reduce exposure to oxidants through a concomitant reduction in the

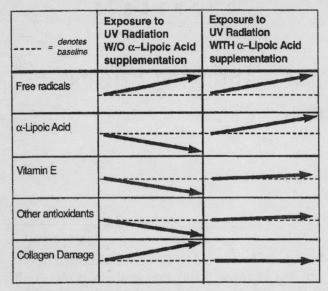

---- = denotes baseline	Exposure to UV Radiation W/O α–Lipoic Acid supplementation	Exposure to UV Radiation WITH α–Lipoic Acid supplementation
Free radicals		
α-Lipoic Acid		
Vitamin E		
Other antioxidants		
Collagen Damage		

(---- denotes baseline.)
Figure 6—Effects to Skin Exposed to UV Radiation With and Without Alpha Lipoic Acid Supplementation.
This figure shows the effects to the skin exposed to UV radiation with and without Alpha Lipoic Acid supplementation. Alpha Lipoic Acid supplementation prevented depletion of Alpha Lipoic Acid and other antioxidants, therefore preventing collagen damage to the skin, which leads to wrinkles and premature "aging."

level of endogenous mutagens produced by normal metabolism. Certainly we can also reduce our exposure to oxidants from external sources in the environment and increase our intake of antioxidant supplements to protect us from undue oxidant damage as well.

Aging is caused by alterations in membranes,

DNA, collagen, chromosomal material, and the proteins, enzymes, and molecules that modulate calcium levels in the intracellular compartments. Calcium regulation also plays an important role in aging and cell death. By sustaining high levels of calcium, we increase oxidative stress—a natural result of the body's response to calcium.

Adverse effects of protein oxidation include memory impairment, and many of the complications associated with diabetes such as neuropathy and cataracts, which are covered in a later chapter.

Cross-linking (which creates destructive, hard, inflexible bonds) is a term commonly associated with aging. Cross-linking at the molecular level causes the body to become stiff and less agile. Large protein molecules, such as collagen in connective tissue, become welded together by cross-links, creating hard, inflexible arteries and wrinkled skin.

The genetic master and copy instructors of all cell functions, the nucleic acids DNA and RNA, can also be cross-linked, causing improper functioning and abnormal cells. These abnormal cells can then cause aging as well as many other conditions, including cancer.

Cross-linking can also be caused by a chemical, acetaldehyde, found in cigarette smoke and smog and made in the liver from alcohol, and by free radicals—destructive entities that are created by radiation and the oxidation of fats, both of which are products of normal metabolism. Free radicals damage proteins, fats, DNA, and RNA. They cause the visible brownish pigment accumulation in skin called age spots.

Free Radicals Implicated in 60+ Diseases

Free radicals are believed to be the cause of destruction and death in nearly all living things. Free radicals can attack, damage, and ultimately destroy any material. They degrade collagen and reprogram DNA and are implicated in more than 60 diseases, including the following:

Adult respiratory distress syndrome

Alcoholism

Alzheimer's disease

Asthma

Cancer

Crohn's disease

Diabetes

Duchenne's muscular dystrophy

Hemoglobin-related disorders

Inflammation

Liver disorders

Neuropathy

Reperfusion injury and ischemia

Varicose veins

AIDS

Allergies

Arthritis (rheumatoid)

Atherosclerosis

Cataracts

Cystic fibrosis

Down's syndrome

Hepatitis

Hypertension

Kidney disorders

Macular degeneration

Parkinson's disease

Stroke

CHAPTER 6

Cancer

Cancer is usually the result of external factors combined with a usually localized genetic predisposition for cancer. The carcinogenic role of free radicals and oxidation is well established through large amounts of research data, which note the involvement of free radicals in the process of cancer initiation and promotion.

There are probably over 100 different ways in which free radicals can cause damage associated with cancer. Carcinogens and many other things, such as radiation (including sunlight), which form free radicals in the body can activate oncogenes which cause cancer.

Free radicals damage fats, proteins, membranes, and DNA. The free radicals may come from external sources such as cigarette smoke, certain hydrocarbons in food, polluted air, and ozone, or internal sources such as from activated neutrophils, prostaglandin synthesis, and many other biological processes.

Free radicals can also damage sensors on cell membranes that regulate cell growth and proliferation. If sensors are damaged, unregulated growth can occur. Unregulated growth and cancer go hand in hand.

Free radicals can damage the genetic material (DNA in the nucleus), causing mutation of the cell. In each cell oxidative damage to DNA occurs at a rate of about 10 times per day (Carney et al.). When the resulting lesions are not perfectly repaired, the cells may mutate. Antioxidants can prevent this damage.

Free radicals can also damage the immune system, which would otherwise recognize and destroy mutated cells before they multiply and become cancerous.

Case Study: Cancer

A 75-year-old man (O.B.) with pancreatic cancer (diagnosed one year previously) came to see me for a consultation. I prescribed a regimen of Alpha Lipoic Acid (150 mg per day), vitamin C (10 grams [10,000 mg] per day), shark cartilage (7,500 mg per day), Essiac™ —an herbal combination of four anticancer agents (4 capsules per day), coenzyme Q-10 (200 mg per day), multivitamins and minerals,* supplemental essential fatty acids,* and Fiber Greens* (see the Appendix).

Following this, he began a course of radiation and chemotherapy for 6 weeks. When I saw him in February 1998, he had regained 10 of the 30 pounds he had lost during chemotherapy. He continues on the prescribed course of supplements. He is physically active without disabling problems.

He continues weekly intravenous chemotherapy without any side effects.

Controversy exists regarding the use of nutritional supplements in patients undergoing chemotherapy or radiation for cancer. Some oncologists believe that nutritional supplements interfere with the therapeutic effects of chemotherapeutic agents. There is a body of evidence, however, that indicates the opposite is true. In practice, we find that cancer patients who are nutritionally supported with high doses of supplements respond better to chemotherapy, with fewer side effects.

Note: Under no circumstances should one self-prescribe the regimins as noted in the case studies recommended by Dr. Sosin and his associates at Whitaker Wellness Center. These are individual situations used as examples. Optimal therapies will vary from person to person. Without a complete medical exam to fully determine one's individual situation, one cannot determine the best course of therapy.

Alpha Lipoic Acid Protects Genetic Material

Alpha Lipoic Acid plays a major role in protecting the genes that determine our health. We know that our family history (our genetics) can increase our susceptibility to certain diseases such as breast cancer, colon cancer, melanoma, and so on. As long as we can prevent this gene from activation, it won't cause any problem. We can do this if certain antioxidants prevent free radicals from reaching the gene.

A gene is a segment of DNA that operates as a

unit within a chromosome to control a specific cell function. There are about 100,000 genes in each of the 46 chromosomes in the nucleus of cells. Genes can reproduce themselves at each cell division, and manage the formation of body proteins through processes called gene expression and regulation. Free radicals and other reactive oxygen species which interfere with normal gene regulation can profoundly influence health and life span.

Genes can be activated by a protein complex within the cell called NF-kappa-B. Oxidation can activate NF-kappa-B, causing it bind to DNA in genes and initiate reproduction. As we grow older, we have higher amounts of activated NF-kappa-B bound to our genes than we did when we were younger.

NF-kappa-B has a negative effect on the immune system, and can also cause defective skin cells and aged skin, as well as defective cells in all the organs, impairing their function throughout the body.

Free radicals, peroxides, and ultraviolet energy can induce the inactive complex to dissociate and allow the NF-kappa-B to penetrate into the nucleus and damage DNA.

Antioxidants Keep NF-kappa-B in Check

The action of NF-kappa-B is controlled by protein subunits called I-kappa-B proteins. When an I-kappa-B protein binds to NF-kappa-B, the complex cannot pass from the cell cytoplasm through the porous two-layered membrane of the nuclear envelope into the nucleus where the genes are located. The goal for health is to prevent the release of excess NF-kappa-

B from the complex, and to permit the body to control its release by normal processes.

Antioxidants inhibit free radicals and other reactive oxygen species and are therefore able to inhibit this activation. Alpha Lipoic Acid is of particular interest because of its ability to work inside the cell. As a relatively very small molecule, it is readily transported through cellular membranes, including the nuclear membrane. It can not only terminate free radicals in the bloodstream and on the cellular membrane, but can also protect NF-kappa-B inside the cell from activation and protect the DNA and genes from damage from certain nuclear factors.

Antioxidants Block Damage from Nitrites

Nitrates and nitrites are common additives in food and cigarettes, but are well known to be carcinogenic (cancer-causing agents) through formation of nitrosamines in the body. These are among the major chemicals in cigarettes believed to cause lung cancer, and are also associated as a causative factor in stomach cancer.

Both antioxidant vitamins C and E have been tested for their ability to prevent tumors from forming in animals due to exposure to nitrites. The antioxidants were as much as 93% effective against tumors forming. Because Alphia Lipoic Acid increases the longevity of these two antioxidants, it can greatly enhance our ability to ward off cancer.

Alpha Lipoic Acid Protects Skin from Cancer and Aging

Skin, as the outermost barrier of the body, is constantly exposed to a variety of oxidative stresses and injury. Topical application of antioxidants is one way to diminish oxidative injury. Alpha Lipoic Acid, as a potent antioxidant which is both fat- and water-soluble, makes an excellent choice to use for skin protection.

Skin cells will convert and release about 25% of the Alpha Lipoic Acid to DHLA. UV radiation is known to deplete the lipophilic antioxidants tocopherol and ubiquinol in skin. Alpha Lipoic Acid was found to significantly protect UV light–induced depletion of ubiquinol by 40% if topically applied 2 hours prior to irradiation (Podda).

Alpha Lipoic Acid and DHLA protect against induced lipid peroxidation and appear to protect special fat-soluble antioxidants in the body which also protect our skin. For example, after administration of Alpha Lipoic Acid to female hairless mice for seven weeks, researchers observed that the levels of the major antioxidants in the skin increased.

UV radiation (both Alpha and Beta gamma rays) is known to cause drastic depletion of these fat-soluble antioxidants. In the Alpha Lipoic Acid–fed animals, some sparing against the loss of these antioxidants occurred. At the end of the irradiation period in the Alpha Lipoic Acid–administered animals, the levels of antioxidants, such as α-tocopherol, ubiquinols, and ubiquinones (i.e., Co-Q-10), were higher than in the skin of controls.

Collagen damage due to oxidative damage in the skin increases between 30 to 40% after exposure to

UVAB radiation. The degree of damage was lower in the skin of the Alpha Lipoic Acid–fed animals both before and after UV radiation exposure. These findings have important implications for skin cancer and skin diseases since depletion of the antioxidant defense mechanism in the skin leads to molecular damage (Packer).

Alpha Lipoic Acid Prevents Radiation Damage

Irradiation is known to produce a cascade of free radicals, and antioxidant compounds have long been used to treat irradiation injury. Alpha Lipoic Acid, but not DHLA, has demonstrated protective effects against radiation injury to sensitive tissues in the body such as the liver, where cells are slow to replace themselves (Kropachova et al.).

The potential benefit of this effect is not only for individuals undergoing irradiation treatment for cancer, but for all of us who are exposed to radiation from the sun. We know that radiation hastens aging of the skin and increases our risk for cataracts, but it is likely to also cause damage in other areas of the body. Unfortunately, it would be almost impossible to do studies for every potential protective benefit of Alpha Lipoic Acid on every area of the body.

Alpha Lipoic Acid Increases Glutathione

In vitro studies demonstrated a dose-dependent increase of 30 to 70% of the glutathione content following Alpha Lipoic Acid administration.

Normal lung tissue of mice also revealed about 50% increase in glutathione upon treatment with Alpha Lipoic Acid. This corresponds with protection from irradiation damage in these in vitro studies (Busse et al.).

Human Studies Confirm Protective Effects of Alpha Lipoic Acid

A recent study examined the effects of 28 days of antioxidant treatment on a variety of blood and urinary parameters in children living in areas affected by the Chernobyl nuclear accident who are continuously exposed to low-level radiation.

- Treatment with Alpha Lipoic Acid alone lowered blood peroxidation values to the same levels seen in non–radiation-exposed children.
- Treatment with Alpha Lipoic Acid with vitamin E further lowered blood peroxidation to below-normal values. Vitamin E alone was without effect.
- Urinary excretion of radioactive metabolites was increased by Alpha Lipoic Acid but not by vitamin E, presumably due to chelation by Alpha Lipoic Acid.
- Liver and kidney functions were also normalized by Alpha Lipoic Acid treatment (Korkina).

CHAPTER 7

Diabetes

Diabetes strikes one out of every 20 Americans. Not only is it the third leading cause of death in the United States, but it also inflicts serious suffering in the form of blindness, nerve damage, heart disease, gangrene, and loss of limbs. In the last 25 years, the incidence of diabetes has increased over 600%, accounting for 300,000 to 350,000 deaths each year during the early 1990s. About half of those with coronary artery disease and three-fourths of those suffering strokes developed their circulatory problems prematurely as a result of diabetes.

Diabetes involves the body's inability to properly metabolize food into energy. The result is a buildup of blood sugar that causes a number of serious problems. With modern-day technology, individuals are able to self-regulate blood sugar to some degree through home glucose tests, medication, and insulin. But even so, normal glucose levels for a diabetic

(180–250 mg per dl) are almost twice the normal range (80–120 mg per dl).

The long-term effects of these elevated blood sugar levels result in oxidative damage (glycation), causing diabetic complications such as cataracts, retinopathy, macular degeneration, stiffened arteries and heart tissue via damaged low density lipoproteins (LDL), and nerve destruction (polyneuropathy). High sugar levels can also result in osmotic changes and reduced blood volume, shock acidosis, coma, and death.

Insulin-dependent diabetes mellitus (Type I) usually results from the body's inability to produce enough insulin, an aftereffect of damage to the beta cells of the pancreas. This form of diabetes usually, but not always, begins in childhood; thus it is often called "juvenile diabetes." This type of diabetes makes up about 10 to 15% of all individuals with diabetes.

Non-insulin-dependent diabetes (Type II) accounts for 85 to 90% of diabetes cases and is usually associated with age and/or obesity. It is sometimes called adult-onset diabetes. Individuals suffering from the disease are able to manufacture plenty of insulin, but the body is not efficient in using the insulin to burn ingested carbohydrates, resulting in elevated glucose levels.

This condition, referred to as insulin resistance, is caused by overweight, improper food choices, lack of exercise, stress caused by illness or injury, and certain medications. This form is caused by insulin resistance of cells or the inability of insulin receptors to utilize insulin efficiently. Usually, diet and oral medication can keep blood sugar levels near normal, but insulin is generally of no value. Type II diabetics generally have high levels of insulin in the blood, but it is ineffective because of the insulin resistance of the tissues.

NADH—Antioxidant Levels Lower in Diabetics

NADH is an enzyme involved in the mitochondrial production of ATP (also known as the Krebs energy cycle). An appropriate supply of NADH is essential to allow certain kinds of reactions to proceed, in this case reactions involving the transport of electrons (or redox reactions).

In diabetic individuals huge amounts of NADH are used for the reduction of glucose to sorbitol. One result of this process is a weakening of the body's ability to detoxify itself. As antioxidants are rapidly used up in detoxification, free radicals and the damage they do spread throughout the body. This is one of the reasons antioxidant levels are so low in diabetics.

Alpha Lipoic Acid Levels Lower in Diabetics

Patients diagnosed with diabetes and many of the complications associated with diabetes such as polyneuritis and atherosclerosis have been found to have lower levels of endogenous (produced in the body) Alpha Lipoic Acid (Altnkirch et al.; Piering et al.). Because higher levels of free radical damage of membrane phospholipids have been shown to be a characteristic of these conditions, there is a great potential benefit of Alpha Lipoic Acid supplementation.

Alpha Lipoic Acid Benefits Diabetes I and II

Alpha Lipoic Acid has potential beneficial effects for both types of diabetes. Most Type II diabetics are hyperinsulinemic; hence, no insulin therapy is warranted. A number of studies have therefore examined other means of increasing glucose uptake. Agents that enhance glucose uptake by skeletal muscles are potentially useful in the long-term treatment of Type II diabetes. Both human and animal studies show that Alpha Lipoic Acid enhances glucose utilization.

Alpha Lipoic Acid Improves Glucose Utilization

Using the obese Zucker rat as an animal model of insulin resistance in obesity, Alpha Lipoic Acid treatment increased the uptake of glucose in the absence or presence of insulin in muscles by over 50% (Henriksen et al.).

In a more recent study by the same research group, lipoic acid increased the uptake of glucose by an average of 78% in lean laboratory rats and by 48% in obese rats. Insulin further enhanced glucose uptake by 30 to 55%. The researchers concluded that Alpha Lipoic Acid works, at least in part, by improving the efficiency of insulin (Henriksen et al.).

Human Studies

In human studies, 1,000 mg of Alpha Lipoic Acid administered intravenously to diabetics enhanced insulin-stimulated whole body glucose disposal by about 50% (Jacob et al.). Supplemental Alpha Lipoic Acid may bring levels of Alpha Lipoic Acid in the body, which are known to be low, back to normal. The various beneficial effects of Alpha Lipoic Acid for diabetics may be due to its reaction with cellular sulfflydryl groups, believed to be involved in the regulation of insulin-stimulated glucose transport. The effect may also be due to the antioxidant function of Alpha Lipoic Acid.

Case Study: Diabetes Type I

M.L., an eighteen-year-old college student, came into the clinic with newly diagnosed insulin-dependent diabetes mellitus. He was complaining of weight loss and the need to urinate frequently. His blood sugar was 600 mg per dl, which is extremely high. The normal range is between 70 and 100. His primary physician had prescribed insulin injections for which the patient required 40 units a day for adequate control of his blood sugar.

We started him on a low glycemic index diet,* and added nutritional supplements including Alpha Lipoic Acid (150 mg per day), the B vitamin, biotin, (8 mg per day), the trace minerals vanadyl sulfate (150 mg per day), chromium (1,000 mcg per day), and a special preparation called Muraglycine®, a cytokine inhibitor which in prior patients has worked to improve glucose control in diabetics.

Within one week his blood sugar level was in the normal

*See the section on the glycemic index, beginning on page 91.

range without the requirement of any insulin. This response has continued much to the surprise of his family. His weight is stable and he feels fine. It is very unusual for insulin to be discontinued in an insulin-dependent diabetic, yet we have seen this response in six out of seven individuals in the last year.

Case Study: Diabetes Type II

F.E., a 67-year-old woman with recently diagnosed diabetes mellitus, came in to see me. Her other physician had started her on Micronase®, a commonly prescribed drug to lower glucose levels in diabetics, but the dose was reduced when dietary changes resulted in a hypoglycemic reaction.

When first seen in our clinic, she weighed 179 pounds and had mild hypertension. I recommended a special diet which eliminated saturated fats, eggs, meat, refined sugar, white bread (only small amounts of whole-grain breads are allowed), pasta, and most starchy foods, including potatoes. I also recommended a daily half-hour walk.

To further lower her blood sugar, I put her on trace minerals chromium (1,000 mcg), vanadyl sulfate (150 mg), biotin (8 mg), the herb gymnema sylvestre (300 mg), and Alpha Lipoic Acid (300 mg) daily.

Gymnema sylvestre increases sensitivity to insulin as well as supports the pancreas to produce insulin.

When seen again four months later, she had discontinued the Micronase® as she was able to control her blood sugar without it through the dietary changes and supplements we prescribed. She had lost nine pounds, her blood pressure was 128/80, and fasting blood sugars were in the normal range of 70–90. Alpha Lipoic Acid and other antioxidants were continued to preclude degenerative processes thought to be mediated by free radicals, including retinopathy, kidney failure, neuropathy, and cardiac disease.

Alpha Lipoic Acid Lowers/Normalizes Blood Sugar Levels

Alpha Lipoic Acid not only normalizes blood sugar levels in diabetics; but also protects against the damage responsible for diabetes in the first place. It has been successfully used in Germany for more than 30 years, where it has reduced the secondary effects of diabetes, including damage to the retina, cataract formation, nerve and heart damage, as well as increasing energy levels. Alpha Lipoic Acid improves nerve blood flow, reduces oxidative stress, and improves distal nerve conduction in diabetic neuropathy.

Alpha Lipoic Acid can terminate free radicals and thus reduce the oxidative stress that can damage the pancreas and cause cataracts, nerve damage, retinopathy, and other side effects. Alpha Lipoic Acid also reduces glycation, which otherwise can damage proteins, especially those of skin and blood vessels. Even more important to diabetics is the fact that Alpha Lipoic Acid, by virtue of its ability to normalize blood sugar levels and the entire glycolysis pathway for conversion of sugar into energy, allows the nerves to recover. Pain is reduced and normal feeling is restored.

Alpha Lipoic Acid increases glucose transport by stimulating the glucose transporters to move from the cell's interior to its membrane—an action done independent of insulin transport. It is believed that the sulfur atoms of Alpha Lipoic Acid are responsible for the translocation. With the restoration of a normal blood sugar level, the number of glucose transporters in the membranes of muscle cells also increase, a most desirable cycle to initiate.

Alpha Lipoic Acid supplementation (300 to 600 mg per day) significantly lowers blood sugar, sorbitol, serum pyruvate, and acetoacetate levels while increasing glycogen (stored energy compound for muscles) in muscles and the liver. At the same time, there is an increase in blood sugar utilization by muscle tissues and a reduction in liver glucose output.

Glutathione and Cysteine Help Normalize Glucose Levels

We know the beneficial effect which Alpha Lipoic Acid has on glutathione and cysteine levels. Both of these amino acids play a critical role in blood sugar regulation.

In Germany, where Alpha Lipoic Acid is currently used as a treatment for diabetic polyneuropathy, researchers made a profound discovery in their efforts to demonstrate Alpha Lipoic Acid's ability to enhance glucose utilization. As insulin resistance of skeletal muscle glucose uptake is a prominent feature of Type II diabetes (NIDDM), these interventions to improve insulin sensitivity could be of tremendous benefit.

One very important Alpha Lipoic Acid study was conducted at the Department of Internal Medicine, City Hospital, Baden, Germany. This study involved 13 diabetic patients who received 1,000 mg of Alpha Lipoic Acid and other diabetic patients, the study "controls" who did not. Both groups were comparable in age, body-mass index, and duration of diabetes, and had a similar degree of insulin resistance at baseline. Administration of Alpha Lipoic Acid resulted in a significant increase of insulin-stimulated glucose disposal. In those patients who took Alpha Lipoic Acid, the metabolic clearance rate for glucose rose by nearly half, whereas patients in the control group did not show any significant change.

This was the first clinical study to show that Alpha Lipoic Acid increases insulin-stimulated glucose disposal in NIDDM. The mode of action of Alpha Lipoic Acid on glucose is not yet completely clear, and its potential use as an antihyperglycemic agent may require further investigation (Jacob et al., 1995).

Caution

Because of these effects of Alpha Lipoic Acid supplementation to insulin-using diabetics on glucose, individuals may require a dose reduction in insulin (or oral antidiabetic medication) to prevent glucose levels from falling too low. Close monitoring of blood glucose levels is required until you have a grasp of how you will respond to Alpha Lipoic Acid supplementation. As a result, caution is advised here.

Alpha Lipoic Acid and Diabetic Complications

One of the most frustrating aspects about dealing with diabetes is the many complications associated with free radical damage. Research has established that the complications from diabetes are directly related to the degree of glucose elevation. Glucose combines with various proteins to form what are called Advanced Glycosylation End Products, or AGES, which then cause deterioration of proteins and of the tissues they comprise. The higher the blood sugar, the more protein degradation occurs. Blood vessels suffer the greatest damage, with accelerated arteriosclerosis affecting circulation to the heart, the brain, the legs, the kidneys, the eyes, and the nerves. Diabetics are subject to heart attacks and heart failure, strokes, leg pains, leg ulcers and amputations, kidney failure, retinal damage, cataracts and blindness, and neuropathic symptoms of tingling, numbness, and pain. The more closely blood sugar is controlled, the less these complications occur.

Another way to prevent complications is to take high doses of antioxidants. Antioxidants block free radical reactions and preserve tissue integrity. It is highly recommended that diabetics take high doses of vitamin E, vitamin C, and other antioxidants such as coenzyme Q-10, pycnogenol, and especially Alpha Lipoic Acid. Insulin-depleted and insulin-resistant diabetics are subject equally to complications, and will benefit from these supplements.

Alpha Lipoic Acid Prevents Glucose-Induced Protein Modifications

Researchers at the University of California, Berkeley, demonstrated that Alpha Lipoic Acid prevents the glycation protein damage associated with elevated glucose levels. When Alpha Lipoic Acid was added, glycation and structural modifications of the protein were significantly prevented. Glycation and inactivation of lysozyme were also prevented by Alpha Lipoic Acid. The researchers concluded that the results suggested a potential for the therapeutic use of Alpha Lipoic Acid against diabetes-induced complications (Suzuki et al., 1992).

Another study at the University of California, Berkeley, to determine the effect of Alpha Lipoic Acid on protein glycation also showed that this substance may play a role in the prevention of diabetic complications by inhibiting glycation and structural damage of proteins. Bovine serum albumin was incubated with glucose in the presence of Alpha Lipoic Acid or DHLA. Both substances inhibited bovine serum albumin glycation (Kawabata and Packer).

German researchers have also demonstrated the protective effect of Alpha Lipoic Acid on membranes with simulation of nondiabetic or diabetic conditions (Hofmann et al.).

Alpha Lipoic Acid Improves Blood Flow, Regenerates Nerves, and Reverses Polyneuropathy

Reduced nerve blood flow due to oxidative stress from elevated glucose levels is a serious problem among diabetics. It is so serious, in fact, that gangrene and the amputation of limbs can be the unfortunate result of failing to reverse the condition. Alpha Lipoic Acid supplementation has clearly demonstrated its capacity to reduce oxidative stress, improve nerve blood flow, and improve distal nerve conduction in diabetic polyneuropathy. This is reviewed in detail in the following chapter.

Case Study: Diabetes, Heart Disease, Neuropathy

T.C. was a 69-year-old man with a history of diabetes mellitus for 27 years. He had been on insulin for the last 17 years. He also had coronary artery disease, with a myocardial infarction two years previously, requiring angioplasty on two vessels. A subsequent coronary angiogram revealed persistent disease, and bypass surgery was recommended but refused. His previous physician had prescribed a nitroglycerin preparation, a beta blocker, and also Coumadin™ because of a recent blood clot in the lungs. Coumadin™ is a blood thinner which works by inhibiting vitamin K activity in the formation of clotting factors. It is also used in rat poisons for the same reason.

Our examination also revealed the absence of reflexes in both legs and reduced vibratory sensation indicative of diabetic neuropathy.

We prescribed a low-fat, high-complex-carbohydrate diet emphasizing foods with a low glycemic index* to improve blood sugar control. To help control his blood sugar and reduce diabetic complications, T.C. was prescribed 300 mg of Alpha Lipoic Acid, vanadyl sulfate, chromium picolinate, biotin, and gymnema sylvestre. L-carnitine, taurine, and coenzyme Q-10 were added to his cardiac regimen. We substituted aspirin for the Coumadin™ and EDTA chelation was initiated to help improve blood flow throughout the body.

When we examined him again eight months later, he had lost 30 pounds in weight. His insulin dose had declined by one third, and his blood sugar control was much better.

*See the section on the glycemic index, beginning on page 91.

We suggested he gradually discontinue his nitroglycerin and beta blocker. He had no chest pains, and a cardiac stress test revealed excellent exercise tolerance. His activity level had improved considerably. He also improved to the extent that he no longer required bypass surgery.

Alpha Lipoic Acid Reduces Elevated Ketones

If the body is unable to use glucose as a source of energy in the body, the body is forced to burn fats instead. This leads to the release of fatty acids into the blood which are converted into ketones, a substance chemically similar to acetone. When an excessive amount of ketones accumulate in the body, it is referred to as ketosis, a potentially serious condition.

Generally, the underlying cause of ketosis is uncontrolled diabetes, in which the lack of insulin prevents glucose from being used as fuel. Symptoms or signs include sweet, "fruity-smelling" breath, loss of appetite, nausea, vomiting, and abdominal pain. If the condition is not treated, confusion, unconsciousness, and death may follow. Ketosis itself is diagnosed by a test that detects ketones in the urine.

The Department of Pediatrics and Child Health, Kurume University, Japan, reported that Alpha Lipoic Acid was found beneficial for a patient, an infant, with elevated ketones. The ketones and other citric acid cycle intermediates had accumulated to such a degree that they were found in combination with a lethal syndrome of metabolic acidosis and renal tubular acidosis. The ketone activity was reduced to between 9 and 29% of control (Yoshida). Alpha Lipoic Acid may have increased the infant's ability to use glucose, restoring normal metabolic activity.

Case Study: Diabetes Mellitus with Multiple Organ Involvement

B.P., a 72-year-old man with a 10-year history of diabetes mellitus, came to see me with a multitude of diabetic complications. He was using 30 units per day of insulin. He was on three medications for control of hypertension prescribed by his previous physician. Diabetes had affected his kidneys, and his renal function had declined to one third of normal, with substantial protein loss as found in his urine. His diabetic retinopathy had progressed so severely that he required laser surgery in each eye. He had severe peripheral neuropathy manifested by pain, tingling, and numbness in his feet. During my examination I found absent reflexes in both legs, with substantial loss of his ability to feel vibrations (termed vibratory sensation). He was also 20 pounds overweight.

I prescribed a primarily vegetarian diet with the exception of fish, which he ate at least twice a week. Supplements included EPA/GLA (6 caps daily), weekly injections of B_{12} (1,000 mcg), and B complex vitamins (100 mg per day). I also prescribed Alpha Lipoic Acid (600 mg daily), and an antioxidant combination formula containing high amounts of antioxidants, carotenoids, and retinal nutrients intended to prevent eye damage.

Six months later his renal function had stabilized, with a decline in urinary protein loss. His neuropathic symptoms of pain tingling, numbness, etc., were gone. The ophthalmologist declared his retinal exam unchanged. The patient had lost 12 pounds, and his blood sugar control was much better.

Usually the complications of diabetes, once started, are relentlessly progressive. This patient experienced improvement or stabilization in his neuropathy symptoms, vision *degeneration, and kidney problems with the help of Alpha Lipoic Acid and other supplements.*

Increased Muscle Energy, Decreased Fat Production

A number of research groups have reported how Alpha Lipoic Acid increases glucose uptake by muscle cells and decreases glucose uptake by fat cells. Dr. M. Khamaisi's group at the University of Negev in Israel reported that the increased glucose transport actually leads to increased energy production. This was confirmed by Dr. Tritschler's group showing increased metabolism and ATP production in muscle tissues, and improved muscle recovery, which permits more work or exercise on the part of the affected individual. The general result is more energy production in muscles and less fat stored in the body (Tritschler). Certainly, these results are of interest not only to diabetics, but to us all!

A Special Note on the Glycemic Index

We often prescribe a diet of foods with a low glycemic index for individuals with diabetes. Glycemic index is a rating system indicating how different foods effect the rise in blood sugar. Foods which have a dramatic effect on blood sugar are rated higher. Reactions are compared to table sugar, which is rated 100, which has the most dramatic effect on sugar levels.

Low glycemic index foods promote a slow, moderate rise in blood sugar and insulin after eating them, which helps keep hunger in check and encourages the body to dissolve body fat by converting it into energy. Low glycemic index foods allow you to consume more calories without gaining weight. They actually increase your metabolic rate.

High glycemic index foods cause sudden, unstable swings in blood sugar, first with rapid, very high sugar and insulin surges, followed by a crash of sugar to excessively low levels. Diabetics (as well as individuals who desire to lose weight and maintain stable energy levels) should *avoid* high glycemic index foods.

In this regard, there are several factors you should never forget:

- Fat, in general, lowers the glycemic rating because it slows absorption. For example, ice cream and yogurt have a lower glycemic rating than non-fat varieties.
- Juiced and pureed fruits and vegetables produce a higher glycemic rating than the whole fruit or vegetable.
- The longer you cook foods like potatoes or vegetables, which are primarily carbohydrates, the more simple the sugars become and the higher the glycemic rating.
- The more you alter a food, the higher the glycemic index rating becomes. Mashed potatoes have a higher rate than whole potatoes. Rice flour has a higher rate than whole rice. In summary, the more intact the food is, the healthier your insulin response will be after eating it.

The following list will help you judge which foods have high and low glycemic index values.

Glycemic Food Value Examples

Low (0–35)

Bread, Pasta, etc.
Coarse whole grain wheat or rye
Pita bread
Cracked or sprouted whole wheat bread
Pasta (all types)
Barley
Bulgur
Buckwheat
Kasha
Couscous
Most beans
Peas
Sweet potato/yam

Dairy
Milk: 1% or skim
Cottage cheese
Buttermilk
Ice milk and ice cream (are high in sugar, but are
    absorbed slower due to their high fat content)
Low-fat artificially sweetened desserts
Yogurt with artificial sweetener
Low-fat artificially sweetened desserts
Low-fat frozen yogurt with artificial sweetener

Fruit
Most fresh whole fruit

Meat/Protein
Shellfish

"White" (low-fat) fish: i.e., cod, flounder, trout, tuna in water
Egg substitutes (cholesterol-free)
Venison
Skinless chicken, turkey, cornish hen (white meat only)

Vegetables
Almost all vegetables

Soups
Low-fat brands: i.e, Health Valley, Pritikin, Progresso, Campbell Healthy Request, and so on

Miscellaneous
Nuts, almonds, walnuts, and so on
Butter
Fructose
Sugar-free gelatin

Medium (36–65)

Bread, Pasta, etc.
100% stone ground whole wheat breads or matzoh
Pumpernickel bread
100% whole grain rye crisp crackers
Brown rice
Boiled or baked potato
Lima beans
Whole corn

Dairy
2% milk
Cheese
Plain yogurt

Fruit
    Natural fruit juices
    Kiwi
    Mango

Meat/Protein
    Higher-fat fish: i.e., salmon, herring
    Lean cuts of beef and pork
    Low-fat cheese
    Eggs

Vegetables
    Beets

Soups
    Most commercial soups (be on guard against soups
        with high fat, high sodium, and starch content.)

Miscellaneous
    Artificially sweetened deserts

High (66–100): Avoid these foods!

Breads
    White bread
    Commercial whole wheat breads
    Commercial rye bread
    English muffins, bagels, commercial matzoh
    Instant, "quick," or precooked grains
    Instant, or one-minute white rice

Dairy
    Low-fat frozen desserts with sugar added
    Low-fat and regular frozen yogurt w/ sugar

Non-fat ice cream and ice milk
Cheese

Fruit
Pineapple
Raisins and other dried fruit
Watermelon
Fruit juice with added sugar or corn syrup

Meat/Protein
Most cuts of beef, pork, or lamb
Hot dogs (including "low-fat" versions)
Luncheon meat
Peanut butter, peanuts

Vegetables
Carrots (high in sugar)
Winter squash (acorn, butternut)

Soups
Powdered or instant soups

Miscellaneous
Glucose and sucrose
Sweeteners: Corn syrup, honey, molasses
Corn starch
Soft drinks
Desserts
Candy

Summary of Recommendations for Diabetics

Eat a low-fat, low-glycemic-index diet.

Avoid animal products except for fish, which should be eaten three or more times a week.

Avoid refined sugars (cakes, cookies, candy, ice cream), fruit juices, and refined grains (bread, pasta, processed cereals). No fried foods. Eat vegetables, especially green vegetables, whole fruits, whole grains (wheat berries, brown rice), beans, nuts, and seeds. Starchy foods, such as pasta and potatoes, should be consumed only in small amounts.

Supplement your diet with the following substances:

Essential fatty acids, (omega-3 and omega-6 fatty acids), most available in ground flaxseeds.

High doses of B vitamins, vitamin C, zinc, selenium, magnesium (at least 500 mg a day), and trace minerals.

Alpha Lipoic Acid (300–600 mg), using higher doses if end organ damage is present, such as in neuropathy or retinopathy.

Additional antioxidants, including coenzyme Q-10 (100 mg), pycnogenol (100 mg), and N-acetyl-cysteine (1,000 mg).

Nutrients to improve insulin sensitivity, including chromium (1,000 mg), vanadyl sulfate (50–150 mg), biotin (8 mg), and gymnema sylvestre (600 mg).

Obtain daily aerobic physical activity, such as walking 30–60 minutes, to increase insulin sensitivity and maintain cardiovascular integrity.

Water, preferably filtered, 2 quarts a day.

Consider these to be toxic: soft drinks, aspartame, caffeine, alcohol if more than one drink per day. Cigarettes are deadly and should be avoided entirely.

CHAPTER 8

Neuroprotective Effects: Neuropathy, Alzheimer's, Parkinson's, etc.

Neuropathy (the painful swelling and destruction of nerve and nerve endings) is a problem commonly associated with diabetes due to oxidative stress. Neuropathy can also result from alcoholism, lead poisoning, or poisoning from certain prescription drugs. Other causes of neuropathies include viral infection and autoimmune disorders, such as arthritis, lupus erythematosus, and periarteritis. Periarteritis is a disease of the small arteries that can lead to hypertension, heart attack, muscle weakness, ulceration of the skin and gangrene, which can require amputation to be performed. In individuals with any of these conditions, higher levels of free radicals accompanied by depressed levels of antioxidants are common.

Oxidative stress may be greater in neurological tissues because of their constant high rate of oxygen consumption and high mitochondrial density. Mitochondria produce free radicals as "by-products" of normal oxidative metabolic processes which damage mitochondrial DNA, creating a free radical cycle of destruction. This vicious cycle may be largely responsible for neurodegenerative diseases as well.

Individuals with polyneuropathy (which simply means there is damage to several nerves in the body) have been found to have lower levels of Alpha Lipoic Acid in their body. Studies have shown that Alpha Lipoic Acid and DHLA as potent antioxidant supplements are effective neuroprotective agents.

Alpha Lipoic Acid Protects the Protectors

The generation of radicals is greatly enhanced during postischaemic reoxygenation. This refers to the restoration of blood flow to the tissues following a heart attack or stroke where blood flow is temporarily interrupted. Our cells are equipped with free radical scavenger enzymes (SOD, peroxidases, catalases) and antioxidants (vitamins C and E, glutathione) to inactivate free radicals. Alpha Lipoic Acid protects and regenerates these important agents through reduction (donation of an electron). The higher the level of antioxidants present and the longer we can keep these antioxidants regenerating, the longer we are protected from oxidative damage.

Alpha Lipoic Acid Reverses Nerve Damage

In March 1995, at an international meeting on diabetic neuropathy in Munich, Germany, several researchers reported the results of clinical studies in which Alpha Lipoic Acid *reversed* the damage of diabetes to the nerves, heart, and eyes of diabetics.

Most of the clinical studies were from European universities and clinics. Study after study reported that Alpha Lipoic Acid safely regenerated damaged nerves. The consensus was that Alpha Lipoic Acid protects through its antioxidant and antiglycemic actions. The meeting concluded that Alpha Lipoic Acid was the agent of choice for the prevention of diabetic complications including neuropathy, cardio-myopathy (a disease of the heart muscle that causes a reduction in the force of heart contractions and therefore in circulation), and retinopathy (disease of the retina of the eye).

Alpha Lipoic Acid Improves Neurological Function—Causes Neurite Sprouting

German studies with high doses of Alpha Lipoic Acid in diabetics have shown that it improves the ability of leg nerves to conduct impulses while improving heart and gastrointestinal functions (Reschke).

Dr. D. Ziegler and colleagues at the Heinrich-Heine University in Dusseldorf, Germany, showed that long-term treatment with Alpha Lipoic Acid induces what is known as nerve "sprouting," that is, the growth of new nerve fibers in a regeneration process. The study showed a significant reduction in pain and numbness in patients in as little as three weeks. The researchers also observed no adverse effects from the high dosage (600 mg per day) of Alpha Lipoic Acid given during the study.

Alpha Lipoic Acid is believed to cause a dose-dependent sprouting of neurites in nerve cells due to improvement in nerve cell membrane fluidity. In animal experiments, Alpha Lipoic Acid promoted nerve regeneration after partial denervation. Alpha Lipoic Acid improves the blood flow in nerve tissues, improves glucose utilization in the brain, and improves basal ganglia function (areas in the cerebrum which are involved in posture and coordination) (Ziegler et al.).

Alpha Lipoic Acid Reduces Neuropathy

In streptozotocin-induced diabetic neuropathy (SDN), nerve blood flow is reduced by approximately 50%, and oxygen deliverance is greatly reduced. The nerve tissue outside the brain is unique in that, compared with nerve tissues inside the brain, glutathione and its related enzymes are reduced to about 10%.

Restored blood flow following a heart attack or stroke (termed *postischaemic reoxygenation*) results in an increase in radicals (hydroperoxides), reduced antioxidant protection, and a breakdown in the blood-nerve barrier. Therefore, the effect to the brain tissue may include swelling and actual tissue death.

Laboratory animals experiencing SDN were evaluated to determine the efficacy of Alpha Lipoic Acid supplementation in improving nerve blood flow, electrophysiology, and indexes of oxidative stress in peripheral nerves affected by SDN. Nerve blood flow was reduced by 50%. At one month after onset of diabetes and in age-matched controls, Alpha Lipoic Acid, in doses of 20, 50, and 100 mg/kg of body weight (a kilogram is 2.2 pounds) was administered five times per week.

The results were as follows:

- Alpha Lipoic Acid did not affect the nerve blood flow of normal nerves, but improved that of diabetic neuropathy in a dose-dependent manner.
- After one month of treatment, Alpha Lipoic Acid–supplemented rats (100 mg per kg) exhibited normal nerve blood flow.
- The most sensitive and reliable indicator of oxidative stress was a decrease in reduced glutathione, which was significantly lowered in induced diabetic and alpha-tocopherol-deficient nerves. The levels were improved in a dose-dependent manner in Alpha Lipoic Acid–supplemented rats.
- The conduction activity of the nerve was reduced in diabetic neuropathy and was significantly improved by Alpha Lipoic Acid, in significant part by reducing the effects of oxidative stress (Nagamatsu et al.).

NOTE: A dosage of 100 mg/kg cannot be used for humans. Rats have a much faster metabolic rate than humans, and because of other differences, we cannot use the same dosage ratio. Most studies show effective dosages for humans for therapeutic treatment of neuropathy closer to 600 mg per day.

The best way to determine the degree of oxidative stress is to look for the degree of reduced glutathione levels, which are significantly reduced in SDN and alpha-tocopherol-deficient nerves. Alpha Lipoic Acid treatment resulted in a dose-dependent improvement in individuals with reduced glutathione in SDN, resulting in normal values for the higher doses in Alpha Lipoic Acid–supplemented rats. The conduction velocity of digital nerves was reduced in SDN and was significantly improved by Alpha Lipoic Acid. Therefore, these studies suggest that Alpha Lipoic Acid improves neuropathy, in significant part by reducing the effects of oxidative stress.

Human Studies for Diabetic Peripheral Neuropathy with Alpha Lipoic Acid

In a three-week randomized, double-blind placebo-controlled human trial, Alpha Lipoic Acid was tested on individuals with diabetic neuropathy. The study used 328 Type II diabetic patients with symptomatic peripheral neuropathy who were randomly assigned to treatment with intravenous infusion of Alpha Lipoic Acid using three different daily doses: 1,200 mg, 600 mg, 100 mg, or a placebo.

Neuropathic symptoms (pain, burning, paraesthesia, which is the uncomfortable "pins and needles" feeling in the skin, and numbness) were scored at baseline and each visit prior to infusion: 0 (increase in symptoms and pain), 2.5 (no change in symptoms and pain), and 5 (significant improvement in symptoms and pain). In addition, a multidimensional specific pain questionnaire (Hamburg Pain Adjective List: HPAL) and the Neuropathy Symptom and Disability Scores were assessed at baseline and day 19. The total symptoms score decreased from baseline to day 19:

- 4.5+3.7 points/Alpha Lipoic Acid: 1,200 mg
- 5.0+4.1 points/Alpha Lipoic Acid: 600 mg
- 3.3+2.8 points/Alpha Lipoic Acid: 100 mg
- 2.6+3.2 points in the placebo

The response rates after 19 days noted improvement in at least 30% of study patients:

- 70.8% in Alpha Lipoic Acid: 1,200 mg
- 82.5% in Alpha Lipoic Acid: 600 mg
- 65.2% in Alpha Lipoic Acid: 100 mg
- 57.6% in the placebo

The total HPAL score was significantly reduced in the 1,200 mg group and 600 mg group as compared with the placebo group after 19 days.

The rates of adverse events were:

- 32.6% in Alpha Lipoic Acid: 1,200 mg
- 18.2% in Alpha Lipoic Acid: 600 mg
- 13.6% in Alpha Lipoic Acid: 100 mg
- 20.7% in the placebo

These findings substantiate that intravenous treatment with Alpha Lipoic Acid at a dose of 600 mg/day over three weeks is the best dose to reducing symptoms of diabetic peripheral neuropathy. The higher dose of 1,200 mg did *not* further improve symptoms but did increase the incidence of side effects. Note also that there were higher adverse effects in the placebo than in the 100 and 600 mg Alpha Lipoic Acid dosages (Gries).

Case Study: Neuropathy

D.S., a 72-year-old woman, was experiencing tingling and numbness in her feet. This was particularly troublesome for her at night and prevented her from sleeping. Her physical examination revealed absent reflexes in her ankles and substantial loss of vibratory sensation. She was treated with our standard vitamin and mineral preparation (called Forward), high doses of essential fatty acids (EPA/GLA, 6 capsules daily), Energy Essentials (2 per day), Fiber Greens (10 caps per day), Alpha Lipoic Acid (300 mgs per day), ginkgo biloba (120 mg), pycnogenol (100 mg), along with intramuscular injections of magnesium, thiamin (vitamin B_1), and vitamin B_{12}, and weekly chelation therapy.

After two months the tingling and numbness had greatly improved. She experienced no sleeping difficulties, and after four months she was virtually symptom-free. She is continuing the same regimen, though at a lower dosage and reduced frequency of chelation.

Neuropathy Can Also Be Due to Drug Side Effects, Excessive Alcohol Consumption, and Lead Poisoning

There are other causes of neuropathy in addition to diabetes. Several drugs which can cause peripheral neuropathy as a side effect include Zerit®, an antiviral agent; cisplatin, an antineoplastic agent; and Flexeril®, a muscle relaxant.

Other causes include dietary deficiencies (particularly B vitamins), persistent excessive alcohol consumption, lead poisoning and metabolic upsets (such as uremia), and autoimmune disorders such as arthritis and lupus. In these disorders, like diabetes, there is often oxidative damage to the blood vessels supplying the nerves.

Alpha Lipoic Acid can benefit neuropathy generally and certainly despite any particular cause. In patients with dietary deficiencies, and alcohol-related neuropathies, B vitamins should be administered as well as Alpha Lipoic Acid.

Alpha Lipoic Acid and the Brain

The brain is subject to problems due to antioxidant stress just like the rest of the body. For example, antioxidant stress can contribute to circulatory problems, with resulting damage to brain cells.

Happily though, Alpha Lipoic Acid can play an important role in brain wellness by virtue of its ability to neutralize potentially toxic substances and oxidants.

Of particular harm to brain cells are the peroxy nitrates, which can destroy the lipid membrane that protects them. Alpha Lipoic Acid has a powerful ability to neutralize peroxy nitrates, disabling their ability to cause harm.

Alpha Lipoic Acid's ability to increase levels of glutathione and other antioxidants is also beneficial for the brain. As glutathione levels diminish, our vulnerability to neurological damage increases. Because glutathione is already poorly absorbed in the intestinal tract, the ability of Alpha Lipoic Acid to increase levels of glutathione in the brain and body is of added significance.

Antioxidants are also known to play a role in the development of neurological disorders such as Alzheimer's, Parkinson's, and Lou Gehrig's disease.

Alpha Lipoic Acid and Memory

Animal studies have shown that Alpha Lipoic Acid is beneficial in helping to restore lost memory in aging subjects, but does not improve memory beyond what is normal in young healthy individuals.

In a study done on mice, Alpha Lipoic Acid (100 mg per kg of body weight for 15 days) improved performance in an open-field memory test. The Alpha Lipoic Acid–treated animals actually performed slightly better than young animals 24 hours after the first test.

Treatment with Alpha Lipoic Acid did not improve memory in young animals, which were already considered normal. The researchers concluded that Alpha Lipoic Acid's free radical–scavenging ability may improve N-methyl-o-aspartate receptor density, leading to improved memory in older individuals.

Alpha Lipoic Acid Increases Cellular Energy Production

In a patient with a deficit of mitochondrial function in both brain and muscle, mitochondria being the major energy-producing component in the cell, Alpha Lipoic Acid was shown to increase the energy availability in general brain and skeletal muscle performance.

In another study, a woman affected by chronic, progressive external ophthalmoplegia and muscle mitochondrial DNA deletion was observed prior to and after one and seven months of treatment with 600 mg of Alpha Lipoic Acid taken by mouth daily.

Prior to treatment, researchers found a decreased

phosphocreatine content in the occipital lobes, accompanied by normal inorganic phosphate level and cytosolic pH. They also found a high cytosolic adenosine diphosphate (ADP) concentration and a high relative rate of energy metabolism together with a low phosphorylation potential. During the post-exercise period, an aspect of the study, the woman's muscles showed an abnormal work-energy cost transfer function and a low rate of phosphocreatine recovery. All of these findings indicated a deficit of mitochondrial function in both brain and muscle.

Treated with 600 mg of Alpha Lipoic Acid daily for 1 month, the woman showed marked improvement in three important areas.

- 55% increase of brain phosphocreatine.
- 72% increase of phosphorylation potential.
- A decrease of calculated ADP and rate of energy metabolism.

After seven months of treatment, MRS data and mitochondrial function had improved further. Treatment with Alpha Lipoic Acid also led to a 64% increase in the initial slope of the work-energy cost transfer function in the working calf muscle and worsened the rate of phosphocreatine resynthesis during recovery.

The patient reported subjective improvement of general conditions and muscle performance after therapy. The researchers concluded that the treatment with Alpha Lipoic Acid caused a relevant increase in levels of energy available in brain and skeletal muscle during exercise (Barbiroli et al.).

Alzheimer's Disease

Alzheimer's disease is a common condition that severely affects both persons with the illness and their families. Alzheimer's disease is a neurodegenerative disorder characterized by loss of memory and progressive decline of cognitive abilities. Although the pathogenesis of this disease is not known and is still under intensive investigation, there are several hypotheses which address certain aspects of the disease. Oxidative stress, for example, encourages antioxidative approaches to secure an effective neuroprotection for the prevention and therapy of Alzheimer's disease. The toxicity of amyloid beta-protein, an amino acid peptide which is associated with plaques in the brains of Alzheimer's patients, seems to be due to oxidative stress in neurons in the brain. It can also be a potential source of free radicals in brain tissue generally.

Studies conducted at the laboratory for Membrane Structure Studies, MCP-Hahnemann School of Medicine, Allegheny University of the Health Sciences, in Pittsburgh, suggest that the biological activity of the Alzheimer's amyloid beta-protein may be related to membrane lipid peroxidation (that is to say, free radical damage) (Walter).

As several laboratory studies suggest that oxidative mechanisms may be involved in the pathogenesis of Alzheimer's, antioxidant nutrients may be useful in disease prevention (Evans and Morris).

Alpha Lipoic Acid is known to prevent cell membrane damage from free radicals. A study at the Department of Pathology, University of Washington in Seattle, utilizing antioxidants which included

Alpha Lipoic Acid, showed that the effects on amyloid beta are enhanced by hyperoxygen (which can cause oxidative damage) and suppressed by hypooxygen and antioxidants, including Alpha Lipoic Acid (Sopher et al.).

Hopefully, more studies will be conducted in the near future to determine how beneficial Alpha Lipoic Acid supplementation would be.

Vitamin E May Help Slow Progression of Alzheimer's

One study showed that vitamin E, combined with the drug selegiline, may slow the progression of Alzheimer's. While it did not provide improvement for the condition, the vitamin-drug mixture slowed the progression of the disease for six to seven months (Sano et al.). Selegiline is an MAO (monoamine oxidase) inhibitor more commonly prescribed for Parkinson's patients as it is believed to have a beneficial effect on L-dopa.

As we have mentioned throughout the book, Alpha Lipoic Acid supplementation supports the levels of other antioxidants including vitamin E and therefore may be a beneficial adjunctive nutrient to help prevent and slow down the progression of Alzheimer's.

Parkinson's Disease

There is some controversy concerning the potential damage of free radicals catalyzed by MAO in neurodegenerative processes. Uncertainty does exist, however, on whether products of oxidation are relevant factors for neuronal cell death in Parkinson's disease. To date, products responsible for impairment of biochemical functions essential for cell viability are not yet identified, and the primary site of damage within the cell is unknown. Ammonia, aldehydes, and hydrogen peroxide are formed via monoamine oxidase–catalyzed oxidations of primary amines. But it is uncertain which of them, if any, is damaging to the cell (Gotz et al.).

Vitamin E May Protect Against Parkinson's

The Rotterdam Study based in the Netherlands investigated whether high dietary intake of antioxidants decreases the risk of Parkinson's disease. All participants were individually screened for parkinsonism and were administered a semiquantitative food frequency questionnaire. The study population consisted of 5,342 independently living individuals without dementia between 55 and 95 years of age, including 31 participants with Parkinson's disease. The participants ingested 10 mg of vitamin E or 1 mg beta-carotene and 100 mg of vitamin E. The data suggested that a high intake of dietary vitamin E may protect against the occurrence of Parkinson's disease (de Rijk).

Glutathione, NAC, and Alpha Lipoic Acid May Protect Against Parkinson's

Researchers have shown that dopamine can trigger an active program of cellular self-destruction, and have proposed that inappropriate dopamine toxicity or its oxidation products may initiate nigral cell loss in Parkinson's disease. Since dopamine toxicity may be mediated via generation of oxygen-free radical species, researchers at the Department of Neurology, Beilinson Medical Center, Petah-Tiqva, Israel, examined whether dopamine-induced cell death in PC12 cells may be inhibited by antioxidants. They found that the thiol-containing compounds [reduced glutathione, N-acetyl-cysteine (NAC), and dithiothreitol] were markedly protective against dopamine toxicity.

The thiol antioxidants (glutathione, Alpha Lipoic Acid, etc.) and vitamin C prevented destruction of dopamine through free radical damage and production of dopamine-melanin. Their protective effect also manifested by inhibiting dopamine toxicity and DNA fragmentation. Intracellular glutathione and other naturally occuring thiols in the body are an important natural defense against oxidative stress. Researchers have found that depletion of cellular glutathione significantly enhanced dopamine toxicity.

The data indicated that the thiol family of antioxidants are highly effective in rescuing cells from dopamine-induced apoptosis and destruction. The researchers stated that further study of the mechanisms underlying the unique protective capacity of thiol antioxidants may lead to the development of new neuroprotective therapeutic strategies for Parkinson's (Offen et al.).

While clinical trials have not yet been conducted, Alpha Lipoic Acid, as a thiol antioxidant, which is known to greatly increase levels of glutathione and other antioxidants, may indeed be very beneficial for individuals with Parkinson's.

CHAPTER 9

Vision: Macular Degeneration, Cataracts, and Glaucoma

The eye is highly sensitive to oxidative damage. Laboratory data show that antioxidant vitamins help to protect the retina from oxidative damage initiated in part by absorption of light.

The retina is the delicate nervous tissue membrane of the eye, continuous with the optic nerve. The optic nerve receives images of external objects and transmits visual impulses through the optic nerve to the brain. The retina is also the portion of the eye which contains the rods and cones.

The exact center, where focus is the best, is referred to as the macula. The macula is the small oval cone-containing area of the retina near the optic nerve. Accurate sight is dependent upon the focus of the image on the macula.

The retina contains a high amount of alpha-tocopherol (vitamin E), vitamin C, glutathione, the carotenoid, lycopene, and other antioxidants as a natural protective mechanism against free radical damage. The

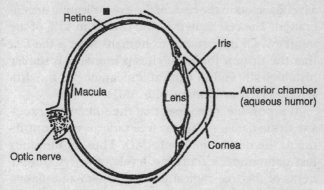

Figure 7—Diagram of the Structure of the Human Eye.

more UV light and other stressors (such as working in front of a computer) that we are exposed to, the faster our stores of antioxidants are used up.

Macular degeneration is the second major cause of blindness in the United States. Animal studies show that retinas containing low levels of carotenoids and vitamin E correspond with early signs of age-related macular degeneration (AMD). The evidence suggests that carotenoids and antioxidant vitamins may help to retard some of the destructive processes in the retina that lead to age-related degeneration of the macula. Research conducted at the Schepens Eye Research Institute, Macular Disease Research Center, and at other institutions, indicates that individuals with low concentrations of carotenoids and antioxidant vitamins and those who smoke cigarettes are at increased risk for AMD (Snodderly; Seddon et al.).

Researchers at the University of California, Davis, examined 62 elderly rhesus monkeys for the presence and severity of macular drusen. Drusen are identified as yellow spots in the back of the eye indicating degeneration. The researchers found drusen in 47% of the monkeys. Of importance to humans here is the fact that the drusen found in rhesus monkeys is similar histologically and in clinical appearance to the drusen observed in humans with AMD.

It is possible, of course, that the sometimes excessive tissue damage done by free radicals may contribute to the development of AMD. Thus, in the study just mentioned, circulating levels of select components of the free radical defense system and plasma thiobarbituric acid reactive substances (TBARS), an estimate of lipid peroxides, were measured. The monkeys diagnosed with drusen were characterized by alterations in concentrations and activities of several components of the free radical defense system. Alterations were most evident with respect to those enzymes associated with copper.

Excessive free radical damage to lipids may be a factor contributing to the occurrence of macular degeneration. This is demonstrated by the findings of higher plasma TBARS concentrations in animals with greater than 10 drusen compared with animals without drusen (Olin et al.).

Higher Serum Levels of Antioxidants Reduce Risk of Macular Degeneration

In a large study with 421 patients and 615 controls with age-related macular degeneration, researchers compared serum levels of carotenoids, vitamins C and E, and selenium. Subjects were classified by blood level of the micronutrient (low, medium, and high).

Persons with carotenoid levels in the medium and high groups, compared with those in the low group, had markedly reduced risks of age-related macular degeneration, with levels of risk reduced to one half and one third, respectively. Although no statistically significant protective effect was found for vitamin C or E or selenium individually, an antioxidant index that combined all micronutrient measurements showed statistically significant reductions of risk with increasing levels of the index. These results suggest that higher blood levels of micronutrients with antioxidant potential, in particular, carotenoids, may be associated with a decreased risk of the most visually disabling form of age-related macular degeneration.

Tocopherols and Carotenoids in Macular Degeneration

Research conducted on antioxidant levels and macular degeneration demonstrate the protective importance of tocopherols and certain carotenoids.

One study group contained a sample of subjects with either retinal pigment abnormalities, the presence of soft drusen, late age-related macular degeneration, or neovascular and exudative macular degeneration. Exudative may refer to hemorrhage (bleeding of the eye) or buildup of serous fluid causing swelling and a multitude of problems. An equal number of controls had no evidence of any of these eye-related problems and were matched with cases by age, sex, and current smoking status.

Average levels of individual carotenoids were similar in cases and controls. Average levels of vitamin E (alpha-tocopherol) were lower in people with exudative macular degeneration. After controlling for levels of cholesterol in the serum, however, the difference here was no longer statistically significant.

Persons with low levels of lycopene, on the other hand, the most abundant carotenoid in the blood, were twice as likely to have age-related macular degeneration. Levels of the carotenoids that compose macular pigment (lutein with zeaxanthin) in the serum, however, were unrelated to age-related macular degeneration.

Very low levels of lycopene, but not other dietary carotenoids or tocopherols, were related to age-related macular degeneration. Lower levels of vitamin E in subjects with exudative macular degeneration, compared with controls, may be explained by lower levels of serum lipids (Mares-Perlman et al.).

While no studies, to my knowledge, have been done on the regenerative effects of Alpha Lipoic Acid on carotenoids, it is likely that it would have this effect as it regenerates other antioxidants such as vitamins E and C, and glutathione.

Cataracts

Cataracts is the term associated with a loss of lens clarity in the eyes and a concomitant impairment of vision. Cataracts form a gray-white film that can be seen behind the pupil. Possible causes of cataracts include:

- Malnutrition
- Amino acid deficiency

- Vitamin deficiency
- Antioxidant deficiency
- Endocrine abnormalities (e.g., diabetes)
- Chemical factors
- Physical factors (e.g., high exposure to UV radiation)
- Accumulation of toxic products (e.g., cadmium from cigarette smoke)

Several studies indicate that high exposure to the sun and other forms of radiation are risk factors for developing cataracts. X rays (gamma, beta, UV and IR rays) pose particularly high risks for developing cataracts. More specifically, while low-level radiation does not induce cataracts, higher-energy radiation does.

Smoking Greatly Increases Cataract Risk

You do not have to be diabetic to suffer from cataracts. If you smoke, you are at risk—it's that simple. Cigarette smoke contains free radicals and leads to a significant increase in the number of free radicals produced. An abundance of research demonstrates that cigarette smoking increases the risk of developing both nuclear sclerosis and posterior subcapsular cataracts. Certainly a greater number of cigarettes smoked per day corresponds with a greater degree of severity in any possible formation of cataracts (Christen, Klein, Shalini, Ramakrishnan, West).

Smoking Increases Cadmium Level, Reduces Vitamin C, Increases Cataract Risk

Cigarettes also increase the risk of suffering heavy metal toxicity from cadmium. We know this by way of the following study. Smokers of three age groups to a maximum age of 58, and who smoked at least 10 cigarettes a day, were compared in terms of cadmium and vitamin C levels to nonsmokers in the same age groups. Researchers found a significant accumulation of cadmium in both the blood and the lenses of the smokers. They concluded that cadmium seems to have a role in the genesis of cataracts in smokers.

In smokers and nonsmokers of two age groups up to a maximum age of 40 and who had no cataracts, researchers found increased levels of cadmium in the blood of smokers only, though the extent of this accumulation was not as great as in chronic smokers in higher age groups.

In both age groups, those up to 50 and those up to 40, the vitamin C content of the lens was on the lower side of normal in chronic smokers and in nonsmokers with cataracts with or without posterior and anterior subcapsular cataracts. There was no significant change brought about by smoking. Blood vitamin C levels were also below normal in smokers and nonsmokers, with and without cataracts (Rarnakrishnan).

We have pointed out this study in light of Alpha Lipoic Acid's capacity to regenerate vitamin C while protecting the body from cadmium toxicity (Muller).

The Role of Oxidative Processes in Diabetic Retinopathy and Cataracts

Several researchers are reporting that the development of the cataract of the eye is an oxidative-degenerative process resembling the physiology of general aging. A measurable parameter here is protein cross-linking or, more generally, the cross-linking and partial loss of function in macromolecules caused by their reaction with aldehydes. One aldehyde in particular, malondialdehyde, a fragment of fatty acid peroxidation, is known to be responsible for the formation of age pigments (lipofuscin) and for lens opacification.

Two types of oxidative processes are thought to occur in tissues exposed to light: (1) activation of oxygen and (2) through activation of pigment molecules (e.g., flavin-containing substances like lutein) which cause the formation of superoxide (O_2) and singlet oxygen. A defect of the protection or repair capacity of the respective tissue results in the observed irreversible damage by these activated oxygen species.

Lens Damage as an Oxidation Process

At the time of birth, approximately 95% of human lens proteins are water-soluble. As we get older, the number of cross-linkages (through free radical damage) increases. The nucleus of the lens assumes an increasingly yellowish color. The oxidation of glycated protein results in the age-dependent accumulation of N-carboxymethyl lysine in the lens. For quite some time it's been assumed that free radical damage to the amino acids tyrosine and tryptophan (molecules which absorb in the ultraviolet range) are responsible for this abnormality.

The cornea of the eye is affected by "characteristic" aging and by ultraviolet light. Degenerative reactions of amino acid (asparagine and glutamine) residues and the degree of hydration of mucopolysaccharides also play a role in lens transparency (Elstner).

Alpha Lipoic Acid Prevents Cataracts

Although cataract formation is a normal complication of diabetes, there is hope, and it goes by the name Alpha Lipoic Acid. Supplementation here decreased cataract formation in a number of trials. For example, Alpha Lipoic Acid prevented the formation of cataracts in vitro in diabetic rat lens cell cultures exposed to high concentrations of glucose. Researchers also observed significant protection of lens ascorbate (vitamin C), tocopherol (vitamin E), and glutathione in the rats given Alpha Lipoic Acid supplements compared to rats not given supplements (Kilic).

Researchers at the University of California, Berkeley, including Dr. Packer, investigated the effect of Alpha Lipoic Acid on cataract formation. They found that in the "cataract-induced" newborn rats, a dose of 25 mg per kg of body weight of Alpha Lipoic Acid protected 60% of the animals from cataract formation.

The "cataract-induced" rats experienced glutathione synthesis inhibition, reduced levels of glutathione, ascorbate, and vitamin E; and developed cataracts. As such, this research becomes a potential model for studying the role of therapeutic antioxidants in protecting animals from cataract formation.

The major biochemical changes in the lens associated with the protective effect of Alpha Lipoic Acid were:

- Increased glutathione
- Increased ascorbate (vitamin C)
- Increased vitamin E levels

Treatment with Alpha Lipoic Acid also restored the protective activities of glutathione peroxidase, catalase, and ascorbate free radical reductase in lenses of the treated animals.

The researchers concluded that Alpha Lipoic Acid may take over some of the functions of glutathione (e.g., maintaining the higher level of ascorbate, vitamin C, and indirect participation in vitamin E recycling). The increase of glutathione level in lens tissue caused by Alpha Lipoic Acid could also be due to its capacity to provide protection for protein thiols. Thus, Alpha Lipoic Acid could be of potential therapeutic use in preventing cataracts and their complications (Maitra et al.).

Dr. Packer of the University of California study hypothesizes that Alpha Lipoic Acid prevents oxidative stress in diabetic conditions by sparing vitamin C. Since vitamin C and glucose share the same carrier in non–insulin-dependent tissues, the elevated blood glucose in diabetes competitively inhibits the cell entry of vitamin C, resulting in localized intracellular vitamin C deficiency.

As a supplement, Alpha Lipoic Acid utilizes other transport systems to enter the cells, is converted to DHLA, and recycles vitamin C. This would explain its positive effects in helping to prevent the formation of cataracts due to diabetes as well as many other complications due to diabetes.

Vitamin C supplementation has been shown to reduce cataract risk. A study found that taking vitamin C supplementation for more than 10 years cuts the risk of early lens opacity—the first sign of cataracts— by 77% and lowers the risk of moderate lens opacity by 83%. Researchers believe that vitamin C helps to saturate the eye tissue (Jacques et al.). Supplementing Alpha Lipoic Acid helps vitamin C to work better and longer.

Alpha Lipoic Acid, Heavy Metals, and Cataracts

In the lens of the eye, elevated glucose is associated with activation of aldose reductase (AR), a precursor to cataracts. Researchers at the Department of Medicine, University College, London, England, demonstrated that Alpha Lipoic Acid inhibited elevated-glucose activation of aldose reductase. The researchers believed that heavy metals may be involved in activating the aldose reductase pathway and that Alpha Lipoic Acid's function as a metal-chelating antioxidant may contribute to its therapeutic role for diabetic complications (Ou).

Case Study: Inflammatory Eye Disease

A. F., a 45-year-old woman, came to us with a one-year history of pain and inflammation in both eyes. She had difficulty reading and was unable to drive a car safely. Her ophthalmologist diagnosed her with uveitis, an inflammation of the outer membrane of the eye. Her ophthalmologist treated her with antibiotics and local steroids, but with minimal results.

We prescribed intravenous infusions with high-dose vitamin C, B vitamins, taurine, and DMSO twice a week. She also started oral Alpha Lipoic Acid in a dose of 900 mg a day, along with a preparation containing carotenoids, bilberry, and other antioxidants. In one month her vision had improved and her reading ability was better. Her ophthalmologist had discontinued her steroids.

After one additional month, her vision was 20/25 in both eyes, her symptoms had fully resolved, and she was able to drive again.

CHAPTER 10

Heart Disease, LDL Cholesterol, and Circulatory Disorders

Free radicals are the primary cause of plaque buildup in the arteries. Oxidation of low-density lipoprotein (LDL) cholesterol (now commonly known as the "bad" cholesterol) damages the arterial walls so they are no longer smooth, presenting an ideal location for plaque to accumulate.

Many studies suggest that antioxidants protect LDL cholesterol against oxidation. As previously mentioned, in addition to providing powerful antioxidant properties itself, Alpha Lipoic Acid recycles other antioxidants in the body such as vitamins C and E. Together they act synergistically as crucial components to warding off free radical damage and maintaining healthy circulation to the heart and throughout the body.

In one study, blood samples of 36 African Americans, ages 16 to 37, showed an inverse correlation between LDL, alpha-tocopherol content, and LDL oxidation rates. LDL samples with higher alpha-tocopherol content exhibit slower LDL oxidation lag rates, demonstrating the ability of Vitamin E to increase LDL resistance to oxidation (Zhang et al.).

The late Dr. Linus Pauling, a two-time Nobel Prize laureate, contended for years that low levels of vitamin C in the blood facilitated cholesterol blockages of the arteries. He showed how high levels protect us in three ways: as an antioxidant, as a healing element for damaged areas of the artery wall before they fill with cholesterol, and as an elevator of high-density lipoprotein (HDL), the "good" cholesterol.

Oxidative Stress Decreased in Coronary Heart Disease Patients with Higher Antioxidant Levels

Antioxidant levels of beta-carotene and vitamin C in blood plasma remain consistent with age, whereas vitamin E levels increase from age 20 up to 59 years, and decrease in individuals older than age 60. Individuals with coronary heart disease, however, show decreased plasma levels of vitamin E accompanied by increased activity of red blood cell SOD, glutathione peroxidase, and catalase (Junqueira).

In a major study from the World Health Organization, which included men and women from 16 different countries, researchers found that a low level of vitamin E in the blood was twice as predictive of a heart attack than either an elevated blood cholesterol level or an elevated blood pressure. Low levels of vitamin E predicted a heart attack 62% of the time while elevated blood cholesterol was predictive 29% of the time and elevated blood pressure only 25% of the time.

Alpha Lipoic Acid Inhibits Lipid Peroxidation

Studies show that Alpha Lipoic Acid can effectively protect liver, brain, skin, and heart tissues against lipid peroxidation (Serbinova). Positive effects here are due largely to the fact that Alpha Lipoic Acid recycles and revives our natural antioxidants such as vitamin E, ubiquinols, and the carotenoids—the major antioxidants that protect the fat-soluble areas such as cell membranes from damage.

Alpha Lipoic Acid Protects Apolproteins Against Oxidative Damage

Dr. Pauling, along with colleague Dr. Matthias Rath, showed that a small particle that resembles LDL cholesterol, called lipoprotein a, or Lp(a) is especially susceptible to free radical damage.

A research team led by Dr. Lester Packer presented the ability of Alpha Lipoic Acid to protect apolprotein against oxidative modification. They demonstrated that with increased Alpha Lipoic Acid antioxidant concentrations, apolproteins were decreased, and the formation of free radical groups inhibited. The results demonstrated that Alpha Lipoic Acid and its derivative, DHLA, are highly efficient in protecting against apolprotein oxidative damage, once again demonstrating its significant effects to ward off heart disease (Yan and Packer).

Alpha Lipoic Acid Prevents Glycation of Hemoglobin and Prevents Iron Oxidation

Hemoglobin is a blood constituent consisting of protein and iron. It is responsible for the transport of oxygen throughout the body. Like all tissues in the body, it is susceptible to oxidative damage. If iron is oxidized, a highly potent radical is produced and circulates in the vulnerable arteries of the body which bring blood and oxygen to all vital organs. Alpha Lipoic Acid prevents this oxidation from occurring (Novak et al.).

Alpha Lipoic Acid Speeds Recovery Following Heart Attack and Stroke—Prevents Free Radical Damage

When there is an interruption in blood flow or oxygen supply to a tissue, it is called ischemia. For example, a heart attack or stroke is precipitated by a blockage in the blood supply to these organs. Reperfusion is the term associated with the administration of drugs to restore blood flow. With reperfusion, however, and as the tissue in question is reoxygenated, a burst of new free radicals follows with possible secondary injury. This is especially important in cardiac tissue (when clot-dissolving drugs for the treatment of heart attack are given) and in the brain.

Agents that prevent ischemia-reperfusion injury may therefore prove important during open-heart surgery, and in the treatment of stroke and other conditions that cause interruption of blood flow.

In a study on rats differentiated by diet, Dr. Packer demonstrated that Alpha Lipoic Acid prevented further cardiac damage following 40 minutes of ischemia and 20 minutes of reperfusion. The mechanical recovery of hearts from the Alpha Lipoic Acid–supplemented group was 68% as compared to 34% recovery of the hearts obtained from rats fed the normal diet.

In addition, Dr. Packer found the content of end products of lipid peroxidation (fluorescence products) after 60 minutes of perfusion was approximately doubled both in the hearts obtained from control animals and in animals given Alpha Lipoic Acid. When hearts were subjected to 40 minutes of ischemia and 20 minutes of reperfusion, fluorescent products increased five-fold. Alpha Lipoic Acid prevented the accumulation of lipid peroxidation products. In this group the content of fluorescence products increased only 2.8 times.

The protective effects of DHLA against rat myocardial ischemia-reperfusion injury are also dependent on vitamin E, suggesting that Alpha Lipoic Acid functions in this system by regenerating tocopherol and decreasing damage caused by free radicals (Haramaki; Serbinova et al.).

Researchers at University of California, Berkeley, also showed that the combination of vitamin E supplementation with DHLA synergistically improves cardiac functional recovery during postischemic reperfusion or posthypoxic reoxygenation of the rat heart. Cardiac levels of glutathione and vitamin E remained significantly elevated with vitamin E and DHLA supplementation. They also showed that the DHLA specifically accelerated the recovery of aortic flow during reperfusion. In addition, DHLA appeared to increase ATP synthesis (energy) in the heart (Haramaki).

Oxidative Stress Elevated in Individuals Who Have Bypass Surgery

Bypass surgery (referring to cardiopulmonary bypass surgery) may be one of the most stressful surgeries ever performed. In 1977 the Coronary Artery Surgical Study (CASS) was done to assess the effectiveness of heart surgery on heart patients. They determined that the risk of dying from the surgery is about three to five times greater than the risk of dying from the disease!

The increased level of oxidative stress resulting from cardiopulmonary bypass surgery and the onset of increased pulmonary vascular permeability is very high. Pulmonary vascular permeability refers to the leaking of fluids due to weakened vascular tissue (usually caused by free radical damage).

Researchers measured and compared risk factors in 10 patients undergoing bypass surgery and 7 normal subjects. Protein accumulation was measured in patients after surgery and in normal subjects as a marker of increased pulmonary vascular permeability. Plasma markers of lipid peroxidation, plasma chelatable iron, total nonheme iron, transferrin, and primary plasma proteinaceous antioxidant activities were measured before and after bypass surgery, and compared with those values found in normal subjects. The following was discovered:

- Protein accumulation was significantly higher in the post-cardiopulmonary bypass patients compared with healthy subjects, indicating pulmonary vascular permeability was significantly increased in patients following bypass. (This also means they were at higher risk for development for elevated homocysteine levels which can create free radical damage to arteries.)

- Concentrations of free radical lipid peroxides were significantly increased following bypass surgery compared to before surgery and to controls.

- Total plasma nonheme iron concentrations before bypass surgery were similar to those concentrations in normal control patients, and significantly increased following surgery.

- Concentrations of transferrin (a protein in the blood needed to move iron from one place in the body to another) were lower in cardiopulmonary bypass patients than in controls and significantly decreased following cardiopulmonary bypass surgery.

- High plasma iron concentrations with a lower level of transferrin were seen following bypass surgery, significantly increased the average percentage of iron saturation of transferrin, increasing from 27.1% to 61.7%.

- Antioxidant levels significantly decreased following cardiopulmonary bypass surgery.

This patient population also had significantly increased plasma markers of lipid peroxidation compared with normal subjects. Cardiopulmonary bypass induced further increases in lipid peroxidation products but a substantial decrease in proteinaceous primary antioxidants. In the majority of patients, there was a significant correlation between the iron saturation of transferrin and the protein accumulation index (Messent et al.).

Other studies researching the effects of free radicals on antioxidants in the heart and on the activity of oxidative mitochondrial enzymes confirm this finding; the heart is highly susceptible to free radical damage following heart attack or bypass surgery. In effect, free radicals depleted the myocardium of antioxidants, leaving the heart more sensitive to the action of oxidative injury (Vaage).

Given this data, the choice is clear: Prior to and following surgery, supplement with high levels of antioxidants including vitamin E, vitamin C, beta-carotene, Co-Q-10, and Alpha Lipoic Acid.

At Whitaker Wellness, of course, we take every possible step to help our patients *avoid* surgery through dietary changes, supplements including antioxidants, magnesium, L-carnitine, TMG, and B vitamins (to help lower elevated homocysteine levels), essential fatty acids, and other lifestyle changes. In three major scientific studies, patients treated with this regimen did just as well as those who had bypass surgery. In a 10-year follow-up, 75% of the patients who had bypass surgery were actually doing worse than the patients treated only with medications we prescribed.

Chelation Helps Eliminate Plaque

At Whitaker Wellness we have much experience using EDTA Chelation, an older but no less admirable therapy for heart and vascular disease. EDTA is a protein-like substance which has an affinity for minerals deposited in the the body. When EDTA is slowly diffused into the body, it attaches to minerals—

particularly heavy metals such as lead, cadmium, and mercury—and makes them soluble. The body then excretes the EDTA-mineral complex through the urine. Because heavy metals tend to lodge in plaque deposits and then encourage their proliferation, eliminating these minerals helps break up the plaque and restore normal circulation.

Alpha Lipoic Acid Is a Metal-Chelating Agent

Alpha Lipoic Acid also acts as a natural therapeutic metal-chelating antioxidant, making it an excellent candidate for the treatment of heavy metals toxicity. Studies show that Alpha Lipoic Acid administration greatly increases the rate of elimination of heavy metals from the body (Grune).

Case Study: Peripheral Vascular Disease, Neuropathy

G.R., a 72-year-old woman, came to us with a history of coronary artery disease. She had bypass surgery performed in 1991. In 1992, during repeat coronary angiography, a laceration of the right femoral artery occurred. In the emergency surgery that quickly ensued, the surgeon placed an aortic bifemoral bypass in her.

By 1996 when she came to us, she had developed increasing numbness and paresthesias (tingling and other abnormal sensations) in her legs, making it difficult to walk more than a short distance. She had other history of hypertension and hyperlipidemia. Our examination revealed weak pulses in the right leg and absent pulses in the left leg, indicating her risk for amputation. She might very well lose her left leg. Reflexes were absent in both knees and ankles, and she had a marked reduction of vibratory sensation.

Further examination revealed very reduced blood pres-

sures in both legs. She agreed to start chelation therapy and an additional therapy called external counterpulsation. In this treatment inflatable cuffs are placed on both lower extremities and around the buttocks. They are expanded under high pressure during the diastolic, or relaxing, phase of the cardiac cycle. They act to increase cardiac output by augmenting blood return to the heart, and to increase blood flow to the lower extremities during systole when the cuffs are deflated. Additionally, she was started on niacin (2,000 mg per day) to lower cholesterol, Alpha Lipoic Acid (300 mg per day), ginkgo biloba (120 mg per day), coenzyme Q-10 (300 mg per day), arginine (1,000 mg per day), and L-carnitine (1,000 mg per day).

Six weeks later her blood pressure had fallen from 190/72 to 130/64. She felt stronger. The tingling and numbness in her legs was much reduced. She was now able to walk over a mile with minimal pain in her calves.

Case Study: Coronary Artery Disease

A.W., a 70-year-old man, came to us with a history of coronary artery disease. In January 1997, his cardiac surgeon performed a five-vessel coronary artery bypass surgery on him. Several months after surgery exertional chest pains recurred. Coronary angiography revealed stenosis at the origin of several grafts. For response, an angioplasty of three grafts was performed. The benefits lasted only two months, however, before chest pains recurred. He was taking aspirin daily, as well as Accupril® for blood pressure control.

He declined any further invasive measures. He had developed a severe leg infection after bypass surgery, requiring prolonged antibiotic therapy.

Standard multivitamins and minerals were prescribed, along with niacin to lower cholesterol, and cardiac supportive nutrients including Alpha Lipoic Acid (150 mg per day), L-arginine (5,000 mg a day), L-carnitine (1,000 mg per day), ginkgo biloba (120 mg per day), taurine (1,000 mg per day), coenzyme Q-10 (300 mg per day), and hawthorne (250 mg per day). He had a course of external counterpulsation, involving timed compressions of the lower extremities and buttocks with pneumatic cuffs. This therapy causes formation of collateral vessels around coronary blockages, and is particularly effective in the treatment of angina following insertion of bypass grafts.

Three months later his chest pain had almost resolved. Treadmill stress testing revealed a 20% increase in exercise time and a 30% increase in cardiac work capacity. Based on these improvements, his prognosis is excellent.

Recent research suggests that coronary artery disease is an inflammatory process, with oxidized cholesterol causing the activation of white blood cells, which migrate into arterial walls and release potent inflammatory chemicals. These chemicals damage the arteries, causing deposits of cholesterol and calcium, and reactive proliferation of smooth muscle cells. Plaques then form which narrow arterial passages. Chest pain occurs due to the decrease of blood flow.

Treatment is directed toward interfering with the oxidation of cholesterol. Alpha Lipoic Acid is a strong antioxidant, and also acts to regenerate vitamin E, an antioxidant proven to reduce the incidence of heart attacks.

Case Study: Heart Disease

Five months previous to his visit to us at Whitaker Wellness, A.M., a 58-year-old man, was admitted to the hospital with severe chest pain. His electrocardiogram was normal, enzyme studies indicated no cardiac damage, and his treadmill stress test was normal as well. He was discharged with a diagnosis of no cardiac disease.

Over the next few weeks he developed typical exertional

chest and arm pressure which resolved with rest. He came to us and repeat stress testing revealed electrocardiographic changes diagnostic of coronary insufficiency. A rapid C-T scan of the heart revealed extensive calcifications of several coronary arteries, consistent with atherosclerosis and with a high risk of future myocardial infarction.

He had a history of mild hypertension and elevated cholesterol, ate an unrestricted diet, did not exercise, and drank 15 cups of regular coffee daily. He was very overweight.

He declined coronary angiography which was recommended by his previous physician, opting instead for an aggressive life-style modification program. He went on a vegetarian diet, omitted coffee, and began a graded exercise program. Nutritional supplements included Alpha Lipoic Acid (150 mg per day), L-carnitine (5,000 mg per day), coenzyme Q-10 (300 mg per day), L-arginine (1,000 mg per day), lysine (1,000 mg per day), garlic (300 mg per day), and Forward (see Appendix).

Within three months he had lost thirty pounds, blood pressure had dropped from 170/100 to 120/65 without medication, cholesterol fell 30 points, and chest pain diminished so that it occurred only with extreme exertion. Repeat stress test and C-T scan of the heart are planned in six months to verify nonprogression of his disease.

Erectile Failure

Impotence, or erectile failure, although a common problem in male diabetic patients, is one of the most neglected complications of diabetes (Chaudhuri and Wiles). Vascular damage, followed by neuropathy, comprise the two most important explanatory factors for the kind of organic erectile dysfunction seen in diabetes. Due largely to free radical damage associated with diabetes, antioxidants such as Alpha Lipoic Acid can suppress the damage, allow the body to repair itself, and restore circulation and erectile success.

Other causes of penile arterial impairment include hypertension, smoking, cardiovascular disorders, alcohol abuse, and age factors (Oka et al.). The damage caused by these factors also directly involves free radicals which antioxidants can help to resolve favorably.

Varicose Veins

Varicose veins (also referred to as chronic venous insufficiency) are not just unattractive abnormally distended veins, but can be very painful and may require surgical ablation or removal (called sclerotherapy).

Valves in the veins prevent blood from draining back down under the force of gravity. Drainage of blood is necessary because veins, unlike arteries, do not have a positive pumping action exerted by the heart or, for that matter, any other intrinsic muscle activity. Venous pumping is performed by the leg muscles massaging the veins during muscular activity. These valves must support a high column of blood and in many people, they often become defective, causing pools of blood to gather in the superficial veins just under the skin. The veins then become swollen, distorted, and unattractive.

Because venous pooling is a situation encountered commonly in varicose disorders, researchers have turned their attention to the potential implications involved—more specifically, researchers assessed oxygen levels in terms of the status of the cells of the vein. When endothelial cells are subjected to reduced oxygen levels, there is an increased synthesis of inflammatory prostaglandins and of PAF (Platelet Activating Factor). This activates leucocytes to release free radicals. The result is local microinflammation, which can become irreversible with painful damage done to the vein by changes in the venous tissue itself (Remacle et al.; Michiels et al.).

Factors which may contribute to the development of varicose veins include the following: obesity, hormonal changes such as during menopause or pregnancy, and standing for long periods of time. In addition, women are affected more often than men, a result perhaps of undesirable shoe style selection or of the constant crossing of legs.

For women, pregnancy of course is a complex time. It is also a time when the potential for varicose veins rises appreciably. Why does this happen? The hormones present during the latter part of pregnancy cause the involuntary muscles in the body to become lax. Thus the most common sites for varicose veins are the back of the calf and anywhere on the inside of the leg. As a result some women experience no discomfort while others experience a severe ache which prolonged standing can make worse.

If surgery is performed to remove a damaged vein, other veins will then assume its function. Sometimes though this is not enough and damaged veins will have to be replaced by other healthy veins in the body. Although this procedure can remove the unsightly dilated vein and improve circulation, it does nothing to help the body to guard against recurrence, which is all too common.

Hemorrhoids Are a Form of Varicose Veins

When we think of varicose veins, we usually think only of those in the legs, but dilated weakened veins can also occur in other parts of the body such as hemorrhoids and esophageal varices (in the esophagus).

"When a vein dilates (opens more than usual) and the valves are damaged, the blood pools in the area causing an unsightly bluish twisted road map pattern just below the skin. Varicose veins in the legs and hemorrhoids can be somewhat avoided by moving more to avoid standing in one place, consuming high fiber foods, and improving the nutritional status of the veins themselves" *(Antioxidants, Your Complete Guide,* by Carolyn Reuben, 1995).

How to Maintain Strong Healthy Veins

- Elevate legs as often as possible to allow gravity to work for you instead of against you.
- Wear comfortable shoes.
- Do upper leg and calf exercises on a regular basis.
- Participate in walking, swimming, and bicycling on a regular basis.
- Flex and extend ankles frequently.
- Increase intake of fiber.
- Utilize antioxidants such as Alpha Lipoic Acid and proanthocyanidins to help decrease free

radical damage and help maintain integrity of the venous structure.

Proanthocyanidins are widely recognized for their ability to provide nutritional support for the strength, permeability, and normal functioning of vascular tissues.

Studies on vascular permeability demonstrate the ability of proanthocyanoside antioxidants to help maintain normal membrane permeability. For example, animals given proanthocyanosides for 12 days maintained normal blood-brain barrier permeability and limited vascular permeability in the skin and the aorta wall.

These results suggest that impairments in leucocyte and granulocyte production of oxygen-free radicals cause capillary plugging and possibly damage to microcirculatory vessel walls in venous disease (Ciuffetti et al.).

In another study, this time on humans, a total of 1,265 patients with age-related diseases such as diabetes, arthritis, vascular disease, and hypertension as well as 1,100 persons in diminished health without apparent disease, were treated with the metal chelator EDTA and antioxidants such as vitamins C and E, beta-carotene, selenium, zinc, and chromium. Good results were observed in the majority of patients. This is encouraging for the initiation of controlled clinical trials (Deucher).

Again, let us recall Alpha Lipoic Acid's special properties: (1) it can provide antioxidant protection against elevated levels of oxidants and (2) it has the profound ability to increase plasma levels of other antioxidants, with which it acts synergistically.

CHAPTER 11

Inflammatory Disorders: Allergies, Asthma, Arthritis, Skin Problems, etc.

Oxidants produced in the body by overactive inflammatory cells, phagocytes, macrophages, and other white blood cells, can increase free radicals by a hundredfold and flood tissue with them, causing localized damage.

Allergies and Antioxidants

Individuals with hypersensitivities are highly susceptible to overactive inflammatory cell activity. The T-suppressor cell is the most sensitive cell of the immune system and the first to be affected by exposure to chemical-free radical pollutants. (Most people don't realize that many substances which irritate allergies (cigarette smoke, smog, pesticides, etc.) are composed largely of free radicals. When hypersensitive individuals encounter irritating substances, their T-suppressor activity diminishes, which in turn increases T-helper cell activity, leading to increased immunoglobulin production and the manifestation of allergy symptoms.

Allergies are difficult to treat because each exposure to the irritating substance further weakens the system, with the creation of even more free radicals. Removal of these chemical pollutants from the body as quickly as possible is essential for effective treatment. Dietary antioxidants can help to reduce the oxidizing effect of the pollutants while acting as conjugators to remove the pollutants from the body (Trevino).

Asthma and Antioxidants

In the last decade we have seen numerous reports of the increased number of asthmatics and asthmatic children. Despite medical advances, there has also been an increase in the number of asthma-related deaths. Higher levels of free radicals due to our industrialized world may be directly correlated with this phenomenon.

Compared to nonasthmatics, asthmatics have a higher level of free radical production generally caused by decreased circulating platelets (red blood cells) and higher levels of white blood cells (neutrophils and macrophages). Platelets are natural inhibitors of the free radical processes in nonasthmatic individuals. In asthmatic patients, however, the free-radical-inhibitory function of platelets decreases.

Antioxidants help normalize platelets in asthmatics by decreasing the presence of white blood cells (neutrophils and macrophages) which are sent in by the body's defense system to combat the "invader," such as cat dander, pollen, mold, and so on.

Case Study: Allergic Rhinitis and Asthma

R.F., an 11-year-old boy, has suffered from allergies and asthma most of his life. He was seen in November 1987 with prolonged and severe exacerbation of cough, wheezing, nasal congestion and discharge. He had not been to school in three weeks, and an unsympathetic grade school principal threatened to expel him from school for the year unless he complied with attendance requirements. His previous physician had prescribed decongestants and steroids and several courses of antibiotics without providing significant improvement.

We eliminated dairy, wheat products, and refined sugars from his diet, and instructed him to acquire a HEPA room air filter. He was prescribed the following supplements: Alpha Lipoic Acid (100 mg daily); quercetin (1,500 mg daily); vitamin C (6,000 mg daily); essential fatty acids EPA/GLA (4 capsules daily); zinc (50 mg daily); and bee pollen (6 tablets daily).

In two weeks he was able to return to school, and after one month his symptoms had almost fully resolved and he was off steroids.

Asthma Attacks Spur Free Radical Production

Oxygen-derived radicals play key roles in allergic inflammatory responses in asthma. These radicals produce many of the pathophysiologic changes associated with asthma and may contribute to its pathogenesis.

Researchers showed that following a severe asthma attack (in animals) the number of white blood cells in lung fluid was increased 3.5 fold compared with nonsensitized but challenged control. They also found that the presence of lipid peroxidation products was 2.4 times higher compared to the controls.

For their part, antioxidant levels were far lower in the lung fluid of the sensitized, challenged animals. The concentration of vitamin E, the major lipid-soluble antioxidant, was 8.7 times lower than that in nonsensitized controls and the reserve of water-soluble antioxidants (thiols and ascorbic acid) was 4 times lower than controls. This indicates an antioxidant/pro-oxidant imbalance associated with an asthmatic episode (Shvedova et al.).

Free Radicals Cause Bronchoconstriction, Increase Mucus and Swelling

Researchers in the Netherlands showed how pulmonary tissue can be damaged in different ways by free radicals formed during inflammation, ischemia reperfusion, or exposure to irritants.

Free radicals induce bronchoconstriction, elevate mucus secretion, and cause microvascular leakage, which leads to edema. Free radicals also create an imbalance between involuntary receptor-mediated contraction and the beta-adrenergic-mediated relaxation of the smooth muscles of the lungs. This increases the risk for spasms and coughing.

Vitamin E and selenium have a regulatory role in this balance between these two receptor responses. The autonomic imbalance might be involved in the development of bronchial hyper-responsiveness, occurring in lung inflammation (Doelman and Bast).

Glutathione Levels Reduced in Asthmatics

In several studies of adults and children with asthma researchers found reduced levels of glutathione peroxidase (Powell et al.; Novak et al.).

The Novak antioxidant study also revealed the impact of asthma on glutathione and the proportion of hemoglobin oxidation products in children. Here, a decreased catalase enzyme activity and a significantly reduced glutathione instability were demonstrated as compared to the controls. Results indicate that antioxidant protection of hemoglobin in asthmatic children is considerably decreased. Hemoglobin, we should recall, is a protein-iron compound in the blood which carries oxygen to the tissues (Novak et al.).

Antioxidants Lessen Damage Caused by Free Radicals

Antioxidants can inhibit the damage caused by free radicals in asthmatic or allergy-prone individuals (Smith).

Vitamin C intake in the general population appears to correlate with incidence for asthma, suggesting that a diet low in vitamin C is a risk factor for asthma. Studies also show the harmful effects of free radical exposure in the children of smokers, resulting in respiratory infections and asthma. Symptoms of ongoing asthma in adults appear to be increased by exposure to environmental oxidants and decreased by vitamin C supplementation. There is also evidence that oxidants produced in the body by overactive inflammatory cells contribute to ongoing asthma.

Vitamin C is the major antioxidant substance present in the airway surface liquid of the lung, where it can protect against oxidants produced within the body as well as oxidants produced within the environment. Nitrogen oxides, which are oxidants that could arise from both endogenous and environmental sources, are protected against by vitamin C, and may be important in the causation and propagation of asthma (Hatch).

Platelet Abnormalities Reduced

In a study whose results were published in 1993, 30 healthy controls and 37 asthmatic patients were observed to determine the effects of platelets on the free radical generation by neutrophils and macrophages and on lipid peroxidation. In healthy individuals, blood plasma poor in platelets (PPP) induced a higher production of free radicals compared to plasma rich in platelets (PRP).

The results obtained demonstrated the inhibitory effect of platelets on free radical generation in asthmatic patients by 1.3–1.2 times.

Antioxidant supplementation inhibited platelets both on free radical (1.4 times) and on lipid peroxidation (1.3 times) and a more marked decrease of neutrophils (1.4 times) compared to patients who did not receive supplementation. The antioxidant preparation potentiates platelet function and accordingly decreases the level of free radicals in blood which prevents inflammation and bronchoconstriction (Boljevic).

Number of Free Radicals Reduced

Fifty-two bronchial asthma patients were studied in regard to generation of active forms of oxygen by leukocytes and of the free radical lipid peroxidation and antiperoxide activity in relation to supplementation with antioxidants. In bronchial asthma exacerbation, free radical production increases compared to the control.

During remission, free radical production decreases but does not reach normal. Bronchial asthma patients receiving antioxidants in addition to the conventional therapy demonstrated a more pronounced lowering of free radical production than those given the conventional therapy alone, providing evidence again in favor of including antioxidants in a combined therapy against bronchial asthma (Daniliak).

Other studies have also demonstrated this beneficial effect of antioxidants. Boljevic found that in patients with steroid-dependent bronchial asthma, the free radical process is more intensive. Regarding the free radical process itself, Boljevic found the most responsive to antioxidant supplementation was aspirin-induced asthma, the mildest exercise-induced asthma. In patients with steroid-non-dependent bronchial asthma and in patients with steroid-dependent bronchial asthma receiving traditional therapy and antioxidants (vitamins E and A and glutamic acid), the decreased free radical generation and decreased effects were greater than in patients not taking antioxidants (Boljevic).

Asthma

Because of the strengths and benefits that we have already seen in Alpha Lipoic Acid, these studies further demonstrate the need for supplementation with Alpha Lipoic Acid not only to regenerate vitamin E and C levels, but also to increase glutathione levels.

Antioxidants Decrease Inflammation

Researchers conducted a study to compare the effects of several different antioxidants, including a thiol group, on individuals with bronchial asthma. They examined respiratory function, hydroperoxides, total and nonprotein thiol groups, and inflammatory and antiinflammatory prostaglandins. All antioxidants were found to lower hydroperoxides (free radicals) and increase the content of thiol groups (group of antioxidants which includes glutathione and Alpha Lipoic Acid). The researchers also noted a rise in the level of anti-inflammatory prostaglandins and a considerable reduction of inflammatory prostaglandins after antioxidant administration (Amatuni). Increased thiol antioxidants were found to decrease free radicals and reduce inflammatory prostaglandins.

Arthritis

Oxygen-free radicals cause tissue degeneration in joint cavities (both forms of arthritis and osteoarthritis). More specifically, the decomposition of hyaluronic acid by free radicals appears to play a role in vivo in the oxidative loss of function of synovial fluid (joint lubricant).

Researchers are now investigating the potential benefit of antioxidant substances for oxygen radicals with inflammatory-associated processes of rheumatic joint disease. For example, several studies have demonstrated antioxidants (1,200 mg alpha-tocopherol) to be safe and effective against arthritis to help improve mobility, reduce pain, and reduce need for additional analgesic medication (Packer).

It is not yet clear, however, if lower levels of antioxidants are the cause or the effect of the disease. Some researchers feel it is possible that antioxidants in the blood mop up free radicals, which are by-products of the inflammation related to the disease (Comstock et al.).

Low Antioxidant Levels Are a Risk Factor for Arthritis

Several micronutrients acting as antioxidants and free radical scavengers have demonstrated protective effects against rheumatoid arthritis.

A case control 20-year study within a Finnish group of 1,419 adult men and women found this intriguing result. In 14 of the individuals who were initially free of arthritis, then developed rheumatoid arthritis; serum alpha-tocopherol, beta-carotene, and selenium concentrations were compared.

Elevated risks of rheumatoid arthritis were observed at low levels of alpha-tocopherol, beta-carotene, and selenium, demonstrating that a low antioxidant level is a risk factor for rheumatoid arthritis years before the disorder is diagnosed (Heliovaara et al.; Comstock et al.).

Significance of Glutathione

Free radicals are trapped by antioxidants such as selenium-containing glutathione peroxidase, which also can inhibit the oxygenation of arachidonic acid to inflammatory prostaglandins and leukotrienes (Honkanen). As we have stated earlier, supplementation with Alpha Lipoic Acid increases concentrations of glutathione in the body, which can be very helpful for individuals with arthritis.

Case Study: Rheumatoid Arthritis:

P.N., a 65-year-old man, had battled against rheumatoid arthritis for many years. Though not disabled, he suffered from aching and morning stiffness in his hands and wrists. He was averse to taking steroids or other anti-inflammatory agents.

Treatment included elimination of wheat and dairy products, and supplementation with Alpha Lipoic Acid (300 mg daily); Fiber Greens (10 capsules daily); essential fatty acids, EPA/GLA (6 capsules daily), glucosamine (1,500 mg daily), chondroitin sulfate (300 mg daily), and niacinamide (1,500 mg daily). Within three months the aching and stiffness were almost gone, his grip strength had increased, and he rarely used pain medications.

Iron Oxidation Aggravates Inflammatory Problems

Researchers in London point out the need for adequate antioxidant levels to protect us from the potential harmful effects of iron oxidation. Iron is an essential mineral involved in the transport of oxygen, in electron transfer, in the synthesis of DNA, in oxidations by oxygen (O_2) and hydrogen peroxide (H_2O_2), and in many other processes necessary to maintain normal structure and function of virtually all mammalian cells.

Without adequate antioxidants, however, to prevent iron oxidation from causing damage, iron oxidation aggravates inflammation through the generation of reactive oxygen intermediates and also through the development of additional free radicals.

Iron oxidation also increases damage associated with hypoxia-reperfusion injury (heart attack and stroke), diseases of the skin (such as psoriasis and allergic hives), and joint diseases (such as arthritis and osteoarthritis) (Morris et al.).

Osteoarthritis

Osteoarthritis, like rheumatoid arthritis, is an age-related disease, in which degenerative changes and superimposed inflammatory reactions (arthritis) lead to progressive destruction of the joints. As we know, cumulative damage to tissues, mediated by reactive oxygen species, has been implicated as a pathway to many of the degenerative changes associated with aging. Appropriate treatment with antioxidants and free radical scavengers is recommended (Henrotin et al.).

In a study published in 1996, researchers hypothesized that increased intake of antioxidant micronutrients might be associated with decreased rates of osteoarthritis in the knees. To test their hypotheses, the researchers made complete assessments of 640 people.

For study participants at the middle level and highest level of vitamin C intake, researchers found a threefold reduction in risk of osteoarthritis progression. This directly related to a reduced risk of cartilage loss. Those with high vitamin C intake also had a reduced risk of developing knee pain. Researchers also found a reduction in the risk of osteoarthritis progression for individuals with an increased beta-carotene and vitamin E intake (McAlindon et al.).

Psoriasis

Individuals with psoriasis (an inflammatory skin condition) also have lower levels of antioxidants. Chronic inflammation, as we discussed, greatly stimulates the production of free radicals, which can further aggravate almost any health situation.

In another study, researchers investigated the red blood cell fatty acid composition and micronutrient saturation of patients with psoriatic arthritis. More specifically, they focused their efforts on determining red blood cell fatty acid composition, selenium status, glutathione peroxidase activity, as well as plasma levels in copper, zinc, vitamins A and E, and thiobarbiturate reactive substances after exposure to an oxidant (H_2O_2). These levels served as an index of susceptibility to lipoperoxidation for 25 patients with psoriatic arthritis and in 25 sex and age matched controls.

Results showed that there was a lower level of the antioxidant selenium in patients with psoriatic arthritis in comparison with controls. Researchers also observed significant direct correlations between red blood cell fatty acids and erythrocyte sedimentation rate, duration of disease, and morning stiffness (Azzini et al.).

As such, this suggests that antioxidant supplementation may benefit individuals with psoriasis and possibly other inflammatory skin conditions.

Case Study: Dermatitis

N.E. was a 68-year-old woman with a 6-month history of a diffuse inflammatory rash covering her entire body. Her skin was fiery red, with induration, thickening, and scaling. She looked like she had been scalded. Prior therapy with steroids and immunosuppressive agents had been ineffective. She was placed on an elimination diet, plus daily nutrients including Alpha Lipoic Acid (600 mg), omega-3 fatty acids (6 g), folic acid (20 mg), zinc (80 mg), vitamin C (10 g), fiber greens, bromelain, and B-complex vitamins. After one month the inflammation started to lessen, the scaling decreased, and the wrinkles were less prominent. Two months later her skin had become smooth and resilient, and the inflammation was present only in blotches. After six months of therapy the rash was gone. She continues on a lower dose of supplements.

Sjögren's Syndrome

Researchers have also determined that female patients with Sjögren's syndrome may benefit from the antioxidant protection of Alpha Lipoic Acid. Sjögren's syndrome is a condition in which the eyes, mouth, and vagina become excessively dry. It commonly accompanies autoimmune disorders such as arthritis and lupus.

Individuals with Sjögren's syndrome suffer free radical damage (in the acinar cells' basal membranes) due to inadequate antioxidant enzyme systems caused by lipid peroxidation reactions (Ron et al.). Again, supplementation with Alpha Lipoic Acid may help to stabilize or to reverse the negative effects caused by the disease on the body's antioxidant enzyme systems.

Crohn's Disease

Patients with Crohn's disease may benefit from the antioxidant protection of Alpha Lipoic Acid as well. Crohn's disease involves inflammation of part of the bowel, usually the ileum, or lower part of the small intestine. It can also occur in the colon.

Case Study: Crohn's Disease

J.M. was a 51-year-old man diagnosed with Crohn's disease 11 years ago. Perianal fistulas developed. Steroids were prescribed twice, and antibiotics on many occasions. When first seen, he was taking an anti-inflammatory agent related to aspirin, and an immunosuppressant drug. He had started taking folic acid, fish oil pills, barley greens, and an herb called cat's claw (una de gato), with improved appetite and a 12-pound weight gain. He had joint pain in his hands, probably related to the Crohn's disease.

He was started on a bowel nutrient preparation, Alpha Lipoic Acid (300 mg daily), coenzyme Q-10, grape seed extract, a fish protein extract, and an increased dose of omega-3 fatty acids. His diet excluded fried and fatty foods, lunch meats, dairy products, chocolate, caffeine, seeds, nuts, sugar, and spices.

Three months later he had gained another 10 pounds, the fistulas had healed, and he was asymptomatic for the first time in years. The immunosuppressant drugs were almost discontinued.

Case Study: Inflammatory Bowel Disease

J.R. was a 19-year-old college student with a 3-year history of inflammatory bowel disease associated with a liver ailment diagnosed as sclerosing cholangitis. Although his bowel disease is in remission, liver enzymes have remained elevated. The natural course of this disease is for the liver inflammation to progress, and for patients to be treated with immunosuppressive agents. He was started on a dairy- and gluten-free diet, using other grains to substitute for wheat. He was also started on a gastrointestinal support regimen utilizing a rice-based concentrate, high doses of omega-3 fatty acids, a fish-derived amino acid supplement, Alpha Lipoic Acid (900 mg per day), and other antioxidants including coenzyme-Q-10, N-acetyl-cysteine, and pycno-genol. One year later he was symptom-free. Liver enzymes remained elevated but did not increase further, and his albumin level, an important indicator of liver function, remained normal.

CHAPTER 12

Alpha Lipoic Acid
and HIV

Acquired immunodeficiency syndrome (AIDS) is caused by infection with a human immunodeficiency virus (HIV). The virus destroys T-cells, white blood cells which play a key role in the immune system to protect us from illness. Compromised immunity makes us more susceptible to illness from a multitude of invasions ranging from candida albicans to cancer.

New drugs have completely changed the way we view HIV and AIDS in the last few years. We now realize that, in many cases, if treated early, a person does not have to die from HIV infection. These drugs are very powerful and do have side effects, such as nausea, diarrhea, and neuropathy, but at least in the case of neuropathy, Alpha Lipoic Acid can help. As explained earlier in the chapter on neuropathy, Alpha Lipoic Acid can help to restore lost nerve function. I know of several HIV patients who had experienced painful tingling and loss of feeling in their feet and toes as a result of the powerful medications they were taking. Depending on the severity of symptoms, improvement can be felt after taking Alpha Lipoic Acid (400–600 mg daily) in 30 to 120 days. Such improvement may take longer in extreme cases, but it is well worth it—some individuals can feel so uncomfortable that it becomes difficult to walk.

Alpha Lipoic Acid can also help the HIV patient directly by preventing replication of the virus through its antioxidant effects, and indirectly by its generalized beneficial effects on white blood cells, including T-cells, which are destroyed by the virus. It is assumed that the higher the viral load in the body, the more difficult it is to maintain T-cells and a necessary degree of immunity.

Antioxidants Enhance Immune Response

Dietary deficiencies of antioxidants can depress immune function through a variety of ways. For example, free radicals can inactivate white blood cells such as neutrophils and macrophages, and other protective agents such as trypsin, which cause inflammatory damage.

Studies show immune enhancement with supplementation of vitamin E and other antioxidants. Higher intakes of antioxidants are associated with lower rates of infection and higher levels of antibodies. As researchers note, HIV-infected patients do have deficiencies in various kinds of antioxidants (Allard, Bendich, Buhl, Dworkin, Bohl).

As a result, it is important for HIV-infected patients to support their antioxidant status. Given the chance, the HIV virus uses free radicals to establish and propagate itself. Free radicals activate HIV replication, and the more antioxidants available to any one person, the harder it is for HIV to grow in that person.

Laboratory studies show intriguing results in this area. For example, if you add antioxidants to a culture dish in which HIV is growing, the antioxidants profoundly reduce activity of the virus, even to the point of inhibiting HIV replication. If the antioxidants are removed, production of the virus increases.

In cultured cells, of course, Alpha Lipoic Acid and dihydrolipoic acid (DHLA) prevent HIV replication and the activation of NF-kappa-B transcription factor, which is regulated by oxidative stress. Remember: Alpha Lipoic Acid converts to DHLA in the body.

For their part, German researchers investigated the effects of Alpha Lipoic Acid supplementation (150 mg three times daily) in 12 HIV-positive individuals. After 14 days, the following results were noted:

- Plasma ascorbate (vitamin C) and glutathione increased.
- Markers of plasma lipid peroxidation decreased.
- T-helper cells increased in 6 patients.
- The T-helper: T-suppressor cell ratio improved in 6 patients (Fuchs).

In cultured cells, Alpha Lipoic Acid and dihydrolipoic acid prevented HIV replication and the activation of NF-kappa-B transcription factor, which is regulated by oxidative stress.

Alpha Lipoic Acid Blocks Replication of HIV-1 and Other Viruses

HIV replication is activated by the release and binding of several factors within the nucleus of the virus itself, specifically, when released, NF-kappa-B attaches to the binding sights on the genetic material (DNA) of the virus. When NF-kappa-B is activated (through oxidation), it binds to the binding sites on the DNA, setting the replication processes in motion.

Remember this, though: NF-kappa-B also regulates a wide variety of cellular and viral genes in addition to HIV. Therefore, oxidative stress can play a role in several additional aspects of HIV infection (Legrand-Poels). Oxidative stress is also involved in immunosuppression (Freed et al.; Aune and Pierce) and tumor initiation and promotion (Cerutti).

Researchers at the University of California, Berkeley, have also demonstrated in vitro that Alpha Lipoic Acid can block replication of HIV and other viruses. They found, in fact, that Alpha Lipoic Acid/DHLA influences the DNA-binding activity of NF-kappa-B (Suzuki).

According to Dr. Packer, human studies at the University of California, Berkeley, with Alpha Lipoic Acid are in the planning stages for the near future.

Alpha Lipoic Acid Blocks Activation of HIV

Scientists have learned how Alpha Lipoic Acid may benefit people with HIV: It inhibits the growth of HIV and inhibits growth more effectively than the much discussed NAC (N-acetyl-cysteine). In in vitro, test-tube experiments, Dr. Packer found that Alpha

Lipoic Acid "completely inhibited activation of a gene in the AIDS virus that allows it to reproduce." It increases the amount of glutathione inside cells, just the place where you need it.

In a recent pilot study of Alpha Lipoic Acid on 12 people with AIDS, glutathione levels increased in 100% of the participants, vitamin C levels increased in 90% of the participants, T4 cells increased in 66%, and other evidence of oxidative stress decreased in over 70%. Unfortunately, no measures of viral load in humans were made. In mice, Alpha Lipoic Acid increases immunity by enhancing the strength of helper T-cells especially. It is capable of finding HIV wherever it is: in lymph cells and neurons (brain cells). A combination of Alpha Lipoic Acid and AZT inhibits reverse transcriptase activity more than either drug alone.

Japanese researchers have also demonstrated the inhibitory effects of Alpha Lipoic Acid against HIV replication, showing that Alpha Lipoic Acid and N-acetyl-cysteine (NAC) significantly depressed HIV-1 reproduction activity (Shoji et al.).

Additional studies have confirmed reports that Alpha Lipoic Acid can block the activation of NF-kappa-B and subsequently HIV transcription, and can be used as therapeutic agents for AIDS.

For example, researchers found that incubation of T-cells with Alpha Lipoic Acid, prior to the stimulation of cells, inhibited NF-kappa-B activation. The inhibitory action of Alpha Lipoic Acid was found to be very potent as only a small amount (4 mM) was needed for a complete inhibition, compared to the 20 mM required for NAC. These results also indicated

that Alpha Lipoic Acid may be effective in AIDS therapeutics (Suzuki).

Alpha Lipoic Acid: Glutathione in T-Cells

Supplemental Alpha Lipoic Acid causes a rapid
increase of intracellular unbound thiols in Jurkat
cells, a human T-lymphocyte cell line. The rise of
cellular thiols is a result of the cellular uptake and
reduction of Alpha Lipoic Acid to DHLA and a rise
in intracellular glutathione. Although the level of
DHLA is 40-fold lower than glutathione, the cellular
concentration of DHLA might be responsible for the
modulation of total cellular thiol levels. Rises in glutathione correlate with the levels of intracellular
DHLA.

Alpha Lipoic Acid had no effect on glutathione
levels when cells were grown in a cysteine-free
medium (an essential amino acid for glutathione synthesis) or after administration of an inhibitor of cysteine synthetase. The rise in glutathione was still
observed after the administration of a protein synthesis inhibitor.

Because of the ability of Alpha Lipoic Acid to
modulate glutathione levels in low dosages, researchers at Stanford University recommended that Alpha
Lipoic Acid administration should be considered as
a potential therapeutic agent in oxidative stress diseases with glutathione abnormalities, including HIV
infection (Han, Derick, and Packer).

Viral Load

As the range of health varies so greatly among individuals who are HIV-positive, an individuals' viral load level may provide an indication of health status. Some individuals carry the virus for 10 or more years before any serious health problems develop (if they ever do). In others, symptoms present themselves a short time after infection. Does this reflect a general state of health and the body's ability to slow replication of the virus?

If supplementation with Alpha Lipoic Acid and other antioxidants can reduce viral load, or slow the virus's replication in the body, the potential benefit could be tremendous indeed. But without research dollars to support large-scale investigations, like many other "natural" unpatentable substances, we may have to "wait and see" what the actual impact will be. This is not an AIDS cure, but it could be a needed support nutrient for immune enhancement for prolonged and improved quality of life. Certainly, Alpha Lipoic Acid supplementation is safe for long-term use in HIV patients.

Case Study: HIV Patient

S.J., a 36-year-old-male, was taking a number of medications to fight HIV including Retrivir (AZT), which is an antiviral, Epivir (antiviral), Viramune (antiviral), Zithromax (antibiotic), Sulfamethoxazole (antibiotic), and Crixovan (protease inhibitor), which was later changed to Virocept. The patient was administered 200 mg testosterone weekly and 200 mg Deca-durabolin weekly. He was also supplementing daily with 600 mg Alpha Lipoic Acid, 3,000 mg vitamin C, 800 IU vitamin E, and 1,000 mg DHA.

At one point his viral load was tested at 125,000 per cubic/ml blood and had only 13 T-cells. At the time of this writing, his viral load is undetectable and his T-cells have increased to over 300 and continue to rise. (Normal T-Cell levels are between 750 and 1,200.) He shows no signs of illness or neuropathy. His weight has remained stable.

Alpha Lipoic Acid Reduces Drug Side Effects

Peripheral neuropathy is a common side effect of many drugs, including some which are commonly prescribed to HIV patients, such as the antiviral agent Zerit®.

The incidence of peripheral neuropathy is dose dependent, meaning the higher the dosage used, the higher the likelihood the side effect will occur. According to the manufacturer, Bristol Meyer, 19 to 24% of patients taking Zerit® require dose modification. The problem occurs because of the drug's effect on mitochondrial synthesis.

Case Study: HIV Patient with Neuropathy

J.R., a 38-year-old male, tested positive for HIV in 1990. He started on AZT for 3½ years with no additional supplementation. His T-cell count dropped from 500 to 200 in this time. Zerit™ was added. After three months he developed peripheral neuropathy and discontinued the Zerit™ due to the discomfort.

Through nutritional counselling he started on Alpha Lipoic Acid, 300 mg twice daily, along with a multiple vitamin, including A, E, and C. The attending physician believed the neuropathy to be too severe to be reversible. After four months the patient experienced a 90% recovery from

162 ALPHA LIPOIC ACID

the tingling and numbness in his fingers and feet. He continued this supplementation as part of this therapy.

In 1998, he remains symptom free with no apparent signs of neuropathy, and a T-Cell count of 300, which is nearing out of the "danger" zone.

Additional Supplements for HIV Patients

Other supplements, especially glutamine, NAC, vitamins C and E, and a healthy overall diet are strongly encouraged not only to slow down replication of the virus, but to help prevent tissue damage through the body from inflammation and other symptoms.

CHAPTER 13

Alpha Lipoic Acid Protects Internal Organs

Alpha Lipoic Acid is presently used in therapy for a variety of liver and kidney disorders. Free radical formation as a part of normal metabolism occurs throughout the body in every organ and gland.

Alpha Lipoic Acid Reduces Kidney Oxidative Stress

There is an excellent chance that kidney damage is due to the damage done by sugar on protein tissues (glycation). This is a common complication of diabetes. As many as 40% of all diabetics eventually develop kidney disease and renal failure, and usually go on dialysis treatment as a result. Homocysteine levels elevate very high in individuals with renal disease, contributing to atherosclerosis. Death due to advanced heart disease is very common at this stage.

The cause of diabetic kidney disease is not completely understood. But we do know this: In part it is due to high amounts of protein breakdown products (proteinuria). Without insulin production, the production of catabolic hormones increases. Overproduction of these hormones causes harmful effects to important proteins and fatty acids in the body. Furthermore, such effects can contribute to ketoacidosis (the excess production of ketone bodies, such as acetone) due to the breakdown of proteins. Excess ketone bodies can overwhelm the system, causing depletion of cations such as sodium. This puts tremendous stress on the kidneys, and the pH of the blood can drop to dangerous levels.

Kidney stress also comes from the effects of elevated glucose levels. When blood glucose levels exceed the "renal threshold" (160–200 mg per dl), additional glucose cannot be reabsorbed and the glucose is excreted in the urine. This also draws water from the cells, which can cause dehydration, leading to thirst, dry skin, and other symptoms.

To examine the protective effects of Alpha Lipoic Acid on the kidneys, researchers artificially induced a higher oxidation level and examined the effects of Alpha Lipoic Acid administration. They first administered an agent (sodium glyoxylate) which increased liver glycollate oxidase radical formation (the major enzyme encouraging free radical formation). This significantly raised the levels of renal tissue calcium and oxalate (reflected simultaneously in their urinary levels). Alpha Lipoic Acid administration had the following effects:

- It lowered oxalate levels in the kidney and urine.
- It decreased glycollate oxidase activity.

The researchers concluded that the possibility of regulating oxalate metabolism with the use of Alpha Lipoic Acid by way of inhibiting liver glycollate oxidase looks promising (Jayanthi).

Alpha Lipoic Acid Prevents Lipid Peroxidation in the Kidneys and the Liver

Researchers at the University of Madras, India, investigated the effects of Alpha Lipoic Acid administration on gentamicin-induced lipid peroxidation in rats. The administration of gentamicin is associated with an increased lipid peroxidation in the kidney. The level of glutathione (GSH) and the activity of three antioxidant systems—superoxide dismutase (SOD), catalase (CAT), and glutathione peroxidase (GPx)—were also decreased in the kidney. The liver, however, did not show any such alterations. Gentamicin plus Alpha Lipoic Acid administration (25 mg per kg) by gastric intubation brought about a decrease in the degree of lipid peroxidation. Researchers also observed an increase in the GSH level and in the activity of SOD, CAT, and GPx. From these observations the researchers concluded that administration of Alpha Lipoic Acid prevents lipid peroxidation, which may, at least partly, play an important role in the cascade of injuries that can result from gentamicin-induced nephrotoxicity (Sandhya).

Case Study: Renal Failure

J.M. was first seen in 1996 with a history of hypertension. Blood pressure was not controlled despite treatment with four antihypertensive medications. She developed progressive renal failure complicated by fluid overload and congestive heart failure, as well as gastroparesis requiring the placement of a gastric feeding tube. Due to progressive weakness, she became bedridden. Biopsy showed the presence of amyloidosis, a degenerative condition which involves the heart, kidneys, digestive tract, and peripheral nerves.

Hemodialysis was started in 1997. Nutritional supplementation, started in 1996, was expanded to include Alpha Lipoic Acid (150 mg daily), plus coenzyme Q-10, glutamine, and other antioxidants.

In spite of her age and debilitated condition, she became gradually stronger, gained weight, started to walk again, and regained gastric function so the feeding tube was no longer necessary. Although adverse reactions to hemodialysis are common in elderly patients with complicated conditions, she had none. Judicious use of supplements can speed the recovery from serious illness, and allow patients to achieve a level of function not otherwise attainable.

Alpha Lipoic Acid Prevents Kidney Stones

Alpha Lipoic Acid has demonstrated the ability to prevent kidney stone formation in laboratory animals. Kidney stones are formed from mineral salts and can cause irritation, organ obstruction and great pain. Increased tissue cholesterol and triglycerides and low phospholipid levels are suggested as risk factors for the development of stones.

Researchers examined the effects of Alpha Lipoic

Acid on altered tissue lipid levels during experimental kidney stone formation. Alpha Lipoic Acid treatment reduced tissue cholesterol and triglyceride levels significantly and raised phospholipids. These alterations were suspected to play a role in the reduced stone formation (Jayanthi and Varalakshmi).

In another study, researchers examined the effects of Alpha Lipoic Acid on certain key carbohydrate-metabolizing enzymes in the tissues of calculogenic rats. The two major enzymes, glucose-6-phosphatase (G6P) and fructose-1-6 diphosphatase (FDP), were significantly inhibited in tissues of calculogenic rats. Alpha Lipoic Acid also reduced the enzyme activities significantly. The citric acid cycle enzymes were not influenced appreciably. The observed alterations are likely to be due to the regulatory effects of oxalate and lipoic acid on the enzyme systems (Jayanthi).

Alpha Lipoic Acid Protects the Liver from Cadmium Toxicity

We know that acute cadmium toxicity causes severe liver disturbances. In this study, isolated rat liver cells were coincubated with Alpha Lipoic Acid or DHLA for up to 90 minutes. Following exposure to cadmium, uptake was diminished with both Alpha Lipoic Acid and DHLA in correspondence to time and concentration. Cadmium-induced damage was decreased as cadmium-stimulated lipid peroxidation decreased.

Alpha Lipoic Acid was not as effective as DHLA as a protectant. Alpha Lipoic Acid increased extracellular acid-soluble thiols different from glutathione. It is suggested that DHLA primarily protects cells by extracellular chelation of cadmium, whereas intracellular reduction of Alpha Lipoic Acid to DHLA provides both intra- and extracellular cadmium chelation/protection (Muller).

Mushroom Poisoning—Elimination of Toxins

Historically, mortality after Amanita mushroom ingestion has ranged from 50 to 90%. Prompt and aggressive therapeutic measures must be instituted quickly to improve the outcome. Successful treatment has been reported using combined therapy of Alpha Lipoic Acid and hemoperfusion (Piering and Bratanow).

Over a period of 15 years, 41 patients with Amanita mushroom poisoning were treated at the University Hospital of Lund, Sweden, where Alpha Lipoic Acid is used in conjunction with other substances for treatment. Treatment consisted of fluid and electrolyte replacement; oral activated charcoal and lactulose; i.v. penicillin, Alpha Lipoic Acid, and silibinin; combined hemodialysis and hemoperfusion in two 8-hour sessions; and a special diet.

The combination of treatment modalities accelerated the elimination of amatoxin from the patients' bodies. The longest period of hospitalization, about 13 days, was required by Group C.

All patients improved and were discharged from the hospital without symptoms. No difficulties were later reported for the majority of those moderately and severely poisoned. The researchers concluded that intensive combined treatment applied in these cases is effective in relieving patients with both moderate and severe amanitin poisoning (Sabeel).

According to some experts such as Dr. Packer, while Alpha Lipoic Acid is often used for therapy in conditions that involve liver pathology, especially mushroom poisoning and alcoholic liver degeneration, there is little evidence that Alpha Lipoic Acid is useful in either of these conditions.

Although case reports describe complete recovery from mushroom (Amanita) poisoning in patients treated with Alpha Lipoic Acid, 10 to 50% of all victims recover without Alpha Lipoic Acid treatment as well (Packer).

Does Alpha Lipoic Acid Protect Us from the Effects of Alcohol?

Several in vitro studies have indicated that Alpha Lipoic Acid supplementation might be beneficial in alcoholic liver disease (Wickramasing). Some researchers, however, feel that these studies suffered from lack of control groups, lack of statistical analysis, or comparative treatments with Alpha Lipoic Acid. In one controlled, double-blind, long-term study, Alpha Lipoic Acid had no effect on the course of alcohol-related liver disease (Marshall). Therefore, its use for the treatment of alcoholic liver disease is not recommended (Packer).

However, it should be pointed out that due to the beneficial effects of Alpha Lipoic Acid on glutathione and cysteine levels and the protective effects against neuropathy, further research may be warranted for Alpha Lipoic Acid as a conjunctive treatment.

Excessive alcohol consumption may also cause a Vitamin B_1 (thiamine) deficiency, which can also cause nerve damage.

Alpha Lipoic Acid Protects Us from Cigarette Smoke

Cigarette smoke contains a number of free radical species. Since many of the diseases caused by smoking involve, at least in part, free radical–mediated processes, it has been proposed that the free radicals in cigarette smoke contribute to smoking-related diseases.

The effects of cigarette smoke on lung fluids have been investigated using plasma as a model system. Supplemental DHLA is protective against cigarette smoke–induced oxidation of antioxidants, proteins, and lipids (Cross).

DHLA also partially protects leukocytes from the damaging effects of cigarette smoke (Tsuchiya). This effect may be due to scavenging of oxidants in the aqueous or lipid phases, or to regeneration of ascorbic acid that has been converted to ascorbyl radical as it is oxidized by cigarette smoke components. In this regard, DHLA could play a role in minimizing the pathological consequences of smoking.

The use of supplemental antioxidants—vitamin

C, beta-carotene, vitamin E, etc.—is widely recognized to be of benefit to smokers. Alpha Lipoic Acid helps potentiate the activity of these, plus offers additional protective benefits against free radical damage.

Alpha Lipoic Acid as a Metal-Chelating Antioxidant

Heavy metals such as iron, copper, lead, mercury, arsenide, and cadmium can be very damaging in the body. Among other problems, they can serve as catalysts for the formation of free radicals in the cells.

As a therapeutic metal-chelating antioxidant, Alpha Lipoic Acid is a good candidate for the treatment of heavy metal poisoning. It may be especially effective against arsenide, cadmium, and mercury. According to one study, Alpha Lipoic Acid administration greatly increases the rate of elimination of heavy metals (Grune).

Other studies are equally promising. For instance, Alpha Lipoic Acid has a profound dose-dependent inhibitory effect upon copper-catalyzed ascorbic acid oxidation and also copper-catalyzed liposomal peroxidation. Alpha Lipoic Acid also inhibits intracellular free radical production of H_2O_2 in erythrocytes challenged with ascorbate, a process thought to be mediated by copper within the erythrocyte (Ou, Tritschler).

Mercury is an environmental contaminant that preferentially accumulates in the kidneys. Researchers at the University of Arizona examined the efficacy of seven chelating agents for the removal of mercury from the kidneys. They found that Alpha Lipoic Acid was more effective than EDTA in mercury removal from kidney tissues (Keith et al.).

Other researchers found that exposure of isolated hepatocytes to Alpha Lipoic Acid or DHLA results in reduced cadmium-induced membrane damage, reduced peroxidation, and reduced depletion of cellular glutathione. These findings were extended to a rat model in which 30 mg of Alpha Lipoic Acid completely prevented cadmium-induced peroxidation in the brain, heart, and testes (Sumathi).

Researchers at the University College London Medical School, suggested that one component of Alpha Lipoic Acid's antioxidant activity requiring study is its direct transition metal-chelating activity. They found that Alpha Lipoic Acid had a profound dose-dependent inhibitory effect upon copper-catalysed ascorbic acid oxidation and also increased the partition of copper into n-octanol from an aqueous solution, suggesting that Alpha Lipoic Acid forms a lipophilic complex with copper ions. Alpha Lipoic Acid also inhibits copper-catalysed liposomal peroxidation.

They also found that Alpha Lipoic Acid inhibited intracellular H_2O_2 production in red blood cells challenged with ascorbate, a process thought to be mediated by loosely chelated copper within the red blood cell. The researchers suggested that prior intracellular reduction of Alpha Lipoic Acid to dihydrolipoic acid is not an obligatory mechanism for an antioxidant effect of the drug, which may also operate via copper chelation (Ou).

CHAPTER 14

Alpha Lipoic Acid for the Athlete

Exercise increases oxidative stress on the body and the need for antioxidant protection. Alpha Lipoic Acid is a very powerful antioxidant. Two studies looking at this effect showed that Alpha Lipoic Acid helps protect red blood cells and fatty acids from both oxidative damage (the type usually experienced from intense training) and UVA damage from intense exposure to sunlight.

This compound has been used in Germany for years as a treatment for diabetes, much like insulin is used in the United States today. A group of doctors from Munich, headed by Dr. Hans Tritschler, reported at an international conference on diabetes that Alpha Lipoic Acid may not only increase glucose uptake by muscle cells but actually decrease glucose uptake by fat cells at the same time. The results of this action may well be more energy production in the muscle and less fat stored in the body.

No tests have yet been performed on healthy, exercising subjects. But it is well established that a large and ever-growing percentage of the American population suffers some degree of insulin insensitivity, especially individuals carrying a substantial amount of excess body fat or those who have diets high in saturated fats (which means most of the population), even though they may not be overweight. If insulin insensitivity is a problem for you and you're trying to build muscle and lose fat, Alpha Lipoic Acid supplementation may help speed recovery, increase endurance, and give you fuller muscles.

Alpha Lipoic Acid looks like the most potent natural insulin mimicker compound on the market, better even than vanadyl sulfate and chromium. Alpha Lipoic Acid may also help enhance the anabolic effects of insulin and may help protect the body against damage from free radicals by working as an antioxidant (100–200 mg taken twice daily).

CHAPTER 15

Alpha Lipoic Acid as a Nutritional Supplement

Alpha Lipoic Acid has been safely used therapeutically to treat diabetic neuropathy for over 30 years at dosages from 300 to 600 mg daily. Even at these high doses, there have been no serious adverse effects reported. No studies indicate any carcinogenic or teratogenic (birth defect–causing) effects.

Alpha Lipoic Acid is absorbed from the diet, transported to the tissues, and taken up by cells, where a majority is rapidly converted to DHLA. Studies show that Alpha Lipoic Acid protects us against deficiencies of vitamins E and C.

Dosage

Supplementation for healthy individuals is usually between 50 and 100 mg daily.

Therapeutic dosages greatly depend on the intent of benefit and severity of one's health situation. As always when a medical problem exists, seek a doctor's guidance before taking any supplement. Because of the improved glucose utilization for diabetics, individuals should monitor blood sugar levels closely to determine possible appropriate modifications in their regimen. If you take too much of it all at once, you could experience low blood sugar levels, which include symptoms such as fatigue, anxiety, jitteriness, confusion, or frustration.

Studies have demonstrated that optimal results for diabetics are achieved with about 600 mg daily (200 mg taken 3 times daily). Better results were not necessarily seen at dosages above 1,000 mg daily; these levels, therefore, are not recommended.

Lethal dosage for humans can be extrapolated from a study done on dogs. In this study, lethal dosage (LD50) is approximately 400 to 500 mg per kg after oral dosing (Packer). As there are 2.2 pounds in 1 kilogram, the lethal dosage for a 150-pound human comes to around 34,000 mg daily (i.e., 34 g, or 681 50-mg capsules). Of course, if you were to take 600 capsules of just about anything, it would probably kill you. Alpha Lipoic Acid is extremely safe.

I have seen timed-release Alpha Lipoic Acid tablets available, but there is no scientific support that shows that these are more advantageous than regular Alpha Lipoic Acid. It is no secret, however, that intravenous or subcutaneous administration of Alpha Lipoic Acid (or most other substances) demonstrates superior utilization by the body compared to oral administration.

Alpha Lipoic Acid supplement forms which claim to provide a slow controlled release into the upper intestine do not have adequate documentation to convince the authors of their benefit. (Dr. Lester Packer concurred, when we asked him about them.)

Side Effects

In humans, the only adverse effects reported to date are possible allergic skin reaction (which is a risk for essentially all foods) and hypoglycemia in diabetics as a consequence of improved glucose utilization with very high doses (AstaMedica).

As Alpha Lipoic Acid may act as an insulin mimicker, if you are diabetic or suffer from insulin sensitivity, you should begin at a low dosage, 50 mg with a meal, eventually working up to a dose of 600 mg per day, taken in divided doses with meals (for example, 200 mg with three separate meals).

As a sulphur-bearing compound, there is a potential risk of adverse effects upon the gastrointestinal tract, and some people using high dosages may experience gas, distension, or a bloated feeling.

Availability

Alpha Lipoic Acid is currently manufactured by only a few companies in a handful of countries including Germany, Russia, Japan, Italy, and China. It can be purchased in many local pharmacies and health food stores, and even on the Internet. Many physi-

cians are also aware of the benefits of Alpha Lipoic
Acid and provide it for their patients. If you feel that
you can benefit from Alpha Lipoic Acid but your
physician is not familiar with its use for your medical
situation, then you can give him or her a copy of this
book.

CHAPTER 16

Resource Guide to Purchasing Alpha Lipoic Acid

Note: This is not a complete list of companies that market Alpha Lipoic Acid, nor is it a "recommended" list.

Capsules and Tablets

Advanced Medical Evolutionary Concepts,
  1-888-367-3432
VitalSource Alpha Lipox, 50 mg and 100 mg

AST Research, 1-800-627-2788
Alpha Lipoic Acid, 200 mg

Baar Nutrition, 1-800-269-2502
Alpha Lipoic Acid, 100 mg

BNG Enterprises, 1-800-445-0161
Natural Treasures Alpha Lipoic Acid, 100 mg

Jarrow Formulas, 1-800-726-0886
Alpha Lipoic Acid, 100 mg tablets and capsules,
300 mg sustained release

JoAnn and David's Health Products, 1-800-700-5402
NOW Formulas Alpha Lipoic Acid, 250 mg

Kal Vitamins, 1-800-669-8877
Alpha Lipoic Acid, 50 mg and 100 mg

Life Extension, 1-800-544-4440
Prolongevity Alpha Lipoic Acid, 250 mg

LifeLink, 1-800-433-5266
UltraPure Alpha Lipoic Acid, 100 mg

Natrol, 1-800-326-1520
Alpha Lipoic Acid, 60 mg, 120 mg, and 300 mg

NatureWorks, 1-212-860-8358
Alpha Lipotene, 580 mg

Nature's Way, 801-489-3631
Alpha Lipoic Acid with Rosemary

Needs Inc., 1-800-634-1380
  Alpha Lipoic Acid: Two available potencies in
  capsule form: 100 mg, 30 capsules per bottle; 300
  mg, 50 capsules per bottle

Olympian Labs, 1-800-473-1663
Alpha Lipoic Acid, 100 mg

SDV Vitamins, 1-800-738-8482
Alpha Lipoic Acid, 50 mg

Schiff,
Alpha Lipoic Acid, 50 mg

Solaray, 1-800-669-8877
Alpha Lipoic Acid, 50 mg and 100 mg

Solgar, 1-201-944-2311
Alpha Lipoic Acid, 60 mg, 120 mg, and 200 mg

Source Naturals, 1-800-777-5677
Alpha Lipoic Acid: Three available potencies in tablet
  form—50 mg, 100 mg, and 200 mg
Alpha Lipoic Acid combined with CO-Q-10: Contains
  30 mg Alpha Lipoic Acid and 30 mg CO-Q-10;
  available in 2 bottle sizes, 30 capsules or 60 capsules

Twinlab,
Alpha Lipoic Acid, 50 mg

Weider Nutrition Group, 1-800-526-6251
Alpha Lipoic Acid

Topical Products

Advanced Medical Evolutionary Concepts,
  1-888-367-3432
VitalSource Skinguard Antiaging Cream

CamoCare, 1-212-860-8358
Hand and Body Lotion, Facial Therapy

CHAPTER 17

Commonly Asked Questions and Answers About Alpha Lipoic Acid

Q: If Alpha Lipoic Acid is called the potato antioxidant, can't we get the benefits by eating a lot of potatoes?

A: Alpha Lipoic Acid is found in potatoes and other foods such as carrots, yams, sweet potatoes, beets, and also red meat, but the amount is so little that supplementation is required to obtain adequate antioxidant protection.

Alpha Lipoic Acid is sometimes called the potato antioxidant because in the 1930s it was discovered that a so-called "potato growth factor" was necessary for growth of certain bacteria. In 1957, the compound was extracted and identified as Alpha Lipoic Acid.

Q: Alpha Lipoic Acid seems like it helps so many different health problems. How can this be so?

A: Antioxidants have the potential to benefit any place in the body susceptible to free radical damage. With over 60 different health problems associated with free radical damage, as an antioxidant, Alpha

Lipoic Acid has the potential to help or prevent any of these conditions.

Q: Because Alpha Lipoic Acid regenerates other antioxidants in the body such as glutathione and vitamins C and E, does this mean we no longer need to supplement these?
A: Studies show that many of these antioxidants actually have a synergistic effect on each other when taken together. Hence, they work better taken together than when taken separately.

Q: What is the best way to take Alpha Lipoic Acid?
A: Because most antioxidants are water-soluble and need to be taken 2 to 3 times a day, and because we know of the synergistic action when taken together, it is best to take it with your other antioxidants.

According to Dr. Packer, "The half life of α-Lipoic Acid in the blood is relatively short, 6 to 8 hours, but I would expect that its life in the tissue would be longer. We have seen some confirmation of this in vitro."

Q: What will I feel after taking Alpha Lipoic Acid?
A: This greatly depends on the individual situation of each person, their health status, and the dosage they are using. In most cases, because it works on a cellular level, you won't really feel anything. Some individuals may feel as if they have more energy.

Individuals with health problems such as diabetes or insulin resistance may experience improvements after a few days in various areas. Some reports indicate that circulation problems and neuropathy may improve after just 30 days. Depending on the severity of your condition, it may take as long as two or three months for you to notice any improvements. Remember this, though: your degenerative condition(s) did not develop overnight, and can't be healed overnight.

Q: Are there any long-term side effects of taking Alpha Lipoic Acid?

A: Taken in the daily dosage range of 20 to 200 mg for average individuals and up to 1,200 mg in individuals with degenerative health problems such as arthritis, lupus, diabetes, HIV, etc., studies do not indicate that side effects are likely. Alpha Lipoic Acid is produced in the body. If you think about it, it seems there would be more adverse effects to *not* taking it.

I spoke to Dr. Packer about the side effects of Alpha Lipoic Acid. He reported that he was not aware of any serious side effects reported at 600 mg taken orally. He pointed out, however, that any substance used to extreme levels can be dangerous. As the toxic dosage here is a very high amount (34 g), Alpha Lipoic Acid seems to be very safe.

I also asked Dr. Packer about the potential pro-oxidant effects if taken in excess. He agreed that antioxidants can turn into pro-oxidants and create free radicals.

For example, UVAB exposure causes vitamin E in the skin to oxidate. But if there is enough vitamin C present to quench the free radicals, it all balances out.

Dr. Packer also pointed out that there are companies that perform tests to measure levels of antioxidants, something you may consider as appropriate.

Q: Some of the effects of Alpha Lipoic Acid seem too good to be true, such as its ability to actually reverse neuropathy. I thought nerve cells and brain cells could not be restored after they die?

A: All cells in the body will renew themselves over and over until the cell becomes damaged and dies. In many cases, new cells form and take their places. This is more evident in areas where cells grow rapidly such as the skin, compared to slow-growing areas (nerve and brain cells, liver cells, bone cells, etc.).

In the case of diabetic neuropathy, where glycation destroys nerve endings, Alpha Lipoic Acid can help prevent further damage from occurring and allow the normal regenerative processes of the body to take place. It is not completely clear how Alpha Lipoic Acid promotes neurite sprouting, or reduces pain, burning, and numbness. Because no other substance has shown such potential, these effects on neuropathy are very encouraging for those individuals suffering from the disease.

Q: If it is so great, why hasn't my doctor heard about Alpha Lipoic Acid?

A: Alpha Lipoic Acid is a nutritional substance naturally found in food and the body (and therefore cannot be patented). Unfortunately, many doctors do not take the time or have the time to educate themselves on the many beneficial nutritional substances available to us.

As a nutritional substance found in nature and manufactured by the body, Alpha Lipoic Acid cannot be patented, meaning anyone can manufacture and sell it. For this reason, U.S. pharmaceutical companies will not invest a great deal of money to educate either physicians or the public on its benefits.

As a result, it is up to each person to learn about the substances that will most benefit him or her. Nutritional science is a great aid here, and a little knowledge can go a long way. For instance, we now need to learn what the body requires to maintain proper balance with a variety of complex nutritionals like DHEA (dehydroepiandrosterone), MCHC (microcrystalline hydroxyapatite), NADH, and Alpha Lipoic Acid!

We cannot rely upon our physician to always know what is best for us. If you are so fortunate to have a doctor who does care enough to do research in nutritional science for you and his or her other patients, you should be grateful. Such doctors are hard to come by.

Q: Could you explain the effects of Alpha Lipoic Acid with regard to HIV?

A: There are two activation sites located on the genetic material of the virus which regulate replication of the cell. These are known as NF-kappa-B binding sites. NF-kappa-B is not just involved in HIV replication; it also regulates replication of other viruses as well as inflammation throughout the body and a wide variety of additional cellular responses. Therefore, this is of importance to individuals with arthritis and other inflammatory conditions.

Oxidative stress is known to activate the transcription process that initiates either replication of the virus or inflammation, etc. Oxidative stress seems to have a negative effect on the immune system as a whole. As Alpha Lipoic Acid has been shown to reduce oxidative stress in the body, the benefits of this substance are clear.

There are also studies showing the positive effect of Alpha Lipoic Acid supplementation on levels of glutathione and cysteine for HIV individuals.

Dr. Packer informed me that researchers at the University of California, Berkeley, are planning in the very near future to further investigate the effects of Alpha Lipoic Acid on individuals with HIV.

Q: Will Alpha Lipoic Acid benefit only individuals who have depressed antioxidant levels?
A: Not necessarily. In many cases benefit level depends on the degree of oxidative stress in the body. The key is to obtain balance between antioxidants and free radicals in the body.

In some situations, Alpha Lipoic Acid has been shown to have effects only in individuals who had depressed levels, such as diabetics in regards to glucose regulation. For the most part, the majority of individuals can benefit from the added antioxidant protection offered by Alpha Lipoic Acid.

Appendix

The majority of patients at Whitaker Wellness Institute are recommended the following supplement preparations:

1. Forward

A multivitamin/multimineral formulated by Dr. Julian Whitaker after years of research on optimal nutritional requirements. Twelve capsules of Forward, the recommended daily dose, provide the following nutrients:

Vitamin A	5,000 IU
Thiamine	50 mg
Riboflavin	50 mg
Niacin	20 mg

Niacinamide . . . . .80 mg
Pantothenic acid. . . . . .50 mg
Pyridoxine . . . . .75 mg
Vitamin B_{12} . . . . 100 mcg
Folic acid . . . . 400 mcg
PABA . . . . .50 mg
Biotin . . . . 300 mcg
Vitamin C. . . . . .2,500 mg
Bioflavonoids. . . . . 100 mg
Vitamin D. . . . . 400 IU
Vitamin E. . . . . 800 IU
Inositol . . . . .40 mg
Choline . . . . 300 mg
Digestive enzymes . . . . .50 mg
Calcium . . . . .1,000 mg
Magnesium . . . . .50 mg
Potassium . . . . .99 mg
Iodine . . . . 150 mcg
Zinc . . . . .30 mg
Copper . . . . 2 mg
Manganese . . . . .10 mg
Chromium . . . . 200 mcg
Selenium . . . . 200 mcg
Molybdenum . . . . 125 mcg
Silica. . . . . .25 mg
Trace minerals . . . . .10 mg

2. EPA/GLA Essentials

Enteric-coated mixture containing the following essential fatty acids per 2 capsules:
Omega 360 mg
Omega-6 fatty acids: 52 mg

3. Energy Essentials

Two capsules per day provide the following:
Magnesium aspartate: 80 mg
Potassium aspartate: 288 mg

4. Fiber Greens Powder or Capsules

A combination of sprouted grain and vegetable powders including apple pectin powder, soya lecithin, vegetable powders, flaxseed meal, alfalfa, barley, wheat grass, acidolphilus and bifidus, and much more.

Bibliography

Achmad, T.H., Rao, G.S., Chemotaxis of human blood monocytes toward endothelin-1 and the influence of calcium channel blockers. Institute of Clinical Biochemistry, University of Bonn, Germany. Biochem Biophys Res Commun 1992 Dec 15;189(2):994–1000.

Ahmad, T., Frischer, H.J., Lab Clin Med 1985 Apr;105 (4):464–71.

Altenkirch, H., Stoltenburg-Didinger, G., Wagner, H.M., Herrmann, J., and Walter, G., Neuroltoxicoll. "Teratol" 12 (1990):619–22.

Amatuni, V.G.; Malaian, K.L.; Zakaharian, A.K., The effect of a single dose of nifedipine, intal, sodium thiosulfate and Essentiale on the blood level of calcium, hydroperoxides, thiol compounds and prostaglandins in bronchial asthma patients. Ter Arkh 1992;64(3):61–4.

Antioxidant status and neovascular age-related macular degeneration. Eye Disease Case-Control Study Group [published errata appear in Arch Ophthalmol 1993 Sep;111 (9):1228, 1993 Oct;111(10):1366 and 1993 Nov;111(11): 1499]. Arch Ophthalmol 1993 Jan;111(1):104–9.

Asta Medica, Alpha Lipoic Acid prescribing information. Asta Medica AG, Frankfurt, Germany.

Aune. T.M., Pierce, C.W. Conversion of soluble immune response suppressor to macrophage-derived suppressor factor by peroxide. Proc. National Academy of Sciences USA (1981) 78: 5099–103.

Azzadnazari, H., Simmer, G., Freisleben, H.J., et al., Cardioprotective efficiency of dihydroAlpha Lipoic Acid in working rat hearts during hypoxia and reoxygenation Arnzmeimittel-Forsch (1993) 43: 425–32.

Azzini, M., Girelli, D., Olivieri, O., Guarini, P., Stanzial, AM., Frigo, A., Milanino, R., et al., Fatty acids and antioxidant micronutrients in psoriatic arthritis. Institute of Medical Pathology, University of Verona, Italy. J Rheumatol 1995 Jan;22(1):103–8.

Backman-Gullers, B., Hannestad, U., Nilsson, L., Sorbo, B., Studies on lipoamidase: characterization of the enzyme in human serum and breast milk. Department of Clinical Chemistry, Faculty of Health Sciences, Linkoping University, Sweden. Clin Chim Acta 1990 Oct 31;191(1–2):49–60.

Baker, J.C., Andrews, P.C., Roche, Recombinant expression and evaluation of the lipoyl domains of the dihydrolipoyl acetyltransferase component of the human pyruvate dehydrogenase complex. Arch Biochem Biophys 1995 Feb 1;316(2):926–40.

Barber, D.A., Harris, S.R., Oxygen free radicals and antioxidants: a review. Department of Surgery, Mayo Clinic & Foundation, Rochester, Minn. Am Pharm 1994 Sep;NS34(9):26–35.

Barbiroli, B., Medori, R., Tritschler, H.J., Klopstock, T., Seibel, P., Reichmann, H., Iotti, S., Lodi, R., Zaniol, P., Lipoic (thioctic) acid increases brain energy availability and skeletal muscle performance as shown by in vivo 31P-MRS in a patient with mitochondrial cytopathy. J Neurol 1995 Jul;242(7):472–77.

Beal, M.F.; Matthews, R.T., Coenzyme Q10 in the central nervous system and its potential usefulness in the treatment of neurodegenerative diseases. Neurology Service, Massachusetts General Hospital, Boston 02114, USA. Mol Aspects Med 1997;18 Suppl:S169–79.

Behl, C., Amyloid beta-protein toxicity and oxidative stress in Alzheimer's disease. Max Planck Institute of Psychiatry, Clinical Institute, Kraepelinstr. 2-10, D-80804 Munich, Germany. chris@mpipsykl.mpg.de Cell Tissue Res 1997 Dec;290(3):471–80.

Behl C., Sagara, Y., Mechanism of amyloid beta protein induced neuronal cell death: current concepts and future perspectives. Clinical Institute, Max-Planck-Institute of Psychiatry, Munich, Federal Republic of Germany. SOURCE: J Neural Transm Suppl 1997;49:125–34

Bendich, A., Antioxidant Micronutrients Annals of the New York Academy of Sciences, Vol. 587, 1990. 168–80.

Boljevic, S., Daniljak, I.G., Kogan, A.H., Changes in free radicals and possibility of their correction in patients with bronchial asthma. Katedra za unutrasnje bolesti br. 2, Prvog medicinskog fakulteta, Moskovske medicinske akademije I. M. Secenov. Vojnosanit Pregl 1993 Jan–Feb;50(1):3–18.

Bolevic, S., Kogan, Daniyak, The antioxidant effect of platelets in the norm and correction of its disturbance in asthmatic patients. Sechenov Moscow Medical Academy, Russia *Oxidants and Antioxidants in Biology*, Oxygen Club of California, Annual Meeting, March 1995.

Bolevic, S., Kogan, S., Grachev, Geppe, Dairova Dinilyak. CO_2 antioxidant effect on the development of asthma. Sechenov Moscow Medical Academy, Moscow, Russia *Oxidants and Antioxidants in Biology*, Oxygen Club of California, Annual Meeting, March 1995.

Buhl, R., Jaffe, H.A., et al., Glutathione deficiency and HIV. Lancet, (1990) 335: 546.

Busse, E., Zimmer, G., Schopohl, B., Kornhuber, B., Influence of Alpha Lipoic Acid on intracellular glutathione in vitro and in vivo. Abteilung fur Hamatologie und Onkologie, Johann Wolfgang Goethe-Universitat, Frankfurt/Main Fed. Rep. of Germany. Arzneimittelforschung 1992 Jun;42(6):829–31.

Byrd, D.J., Krohn, H.P., Winkler, L., Steinborn, C., Hadam, M., Brodehl, J., Neonatal pyruvate dehydrogenase deficiency with lipoic acid responsive lactic acidaemia and hyperammonaemia. Eur J Pediatr 1989 Apr;148(6):543–47.

Carney, J.M., et al., Reversal of age-related increase in brain protein osidation, decrease in enzyme activity, and loss in temporal and spatial memory by chronic administration of the spin trapping compound N-tertbutyl-a-phenyl-nitrone. Proc Natl Acad Aci 1991:88: 3633–36.

Cassarino, D.S., Fall, C.P., Swerdlow, R.H., Smith, T.S., Halvorsen, E.M., Miller, S.W., Parks, J.P., Parker, W.D., Jr., Bennett, J.P., Jr., Elevated reactive oxygen species and antioxidant enzyme activities in animal and cellular models of Parkinson's disease. The Neuroscience Program, University of Virginia Health Sciences Center, Charlottesville 22908, USA.: Biochim Biophys Acta 1997 Nov 28; 1362(1):77–86.

Ceballos-Picot, I., Berr, C., Legrain, S., Hellier, G., Thevenin, M., Nicole, A., Merad-Boudia, M., Peripheral antioxidant enzyme activities and selenium in elderly subjects and in dementia of Alzheimer's type—place of the extracellular glutathione peroxidase. Department of Biochemistry B and A, Necker Hospital, Paris, France. Free Radic Biol Med 1996;20(4):579–87.

Chaudhuri, A., Wiles, P., Optimal treatment of erectile failure in patients with diabetes. Diabetes Centre, North Manchester Healthcare NHS Trust, Crumpsall, England. Drugs 1995 Apr;49(4):548–54.

Chen, C., Loo, G., Inhibition of lecithin: cholesterol acyltransferase activity in human blood plasma by cigarette smoke extract and reactivealdehydes. J Biochem Toxicol 1995 Jun;10(3):121–28.

Christen, W.G,. Manson, J.E., Seddon, J.M,. Glynn, R.J,. Buring, J.E., Rosner, B., Hennekens, C.H., A prospective study of cigarette smoking and risk of cataract in men. Channing Laboratory, Department of Medicine, Harvard Medical School, Boston, MA. JAMA 1992 Aug 26;268 (8):989–93.

Ciuffetti, G., Mannarino, E., Paltriccia, R., Malagigi, V., Sergi, F., Paulisch, P., Pasqualini, L., Lupattelli, G., Leuco-cyte activity in chronic venous insufficiency. Dept. of Internal Medicine, Pathology and Pharmacology, University of Perugia, Italy. Int Angiol 1994 Dec;13(4):312–16.

Cohen-Addad, C., Pares, S., Sieker, L., Neuburger, M., Douce, R., The lipoamide arm in the glycine decarboxylase complex is not freely swinging. Nat Struct Biol 1995 Jan;2(1):63–68.

Comstock, G., et al., Annals of Rheumatic Diseases, 1997, 56: 323–25.

Constantinescu, A., Pick, U., Handelman, G.J., Haramaki, N., Han, D., Podda, M., Tritschler, H.J., Packer, L., Reduction and transport of Alpha Lipoic Acid by human erythro-cytes. Biochem Pharmacol 1995 Jul 17;50(2):253–61. [a]

Constantinescu, A., Tritschler, H., Packer, L., Alpha Lipoic Acid protects against hemolysis of human erythrocytes induced by peroxyl radicals. The azo initiator of peroxyl radicals 2,2'-azobis Biochem Mol Biol Int 1994 Jul;33(4):669–79. [b]

Culter, R.G., Carotenoids and retinol; their possible importance in determining longevity of primate species. Proc Natl Acad Science, 1984, 81, pp. 7627–31. [a]

Culter, R.G., Peroxide-producing potential of tissues: inverse coorelation with longevity of mammalian species. Pro Natl Acad Sciences, 1985,82, pp. 4798–802. [b]

Daniliak, I.G., Kogan, A.K., Bolevich, S., The generation of active forms of oxygen by the blood leukocytes, lipid peroxidation and antiperoxide protection in bronchial asthma patients. Ter Arkh 1992;64(3):54–57.

Deucher, G., Antioxidant therapy in the aging process. Clinica Guilherme Paulo Deucher, São Paulo, Brazil. EXS 1992;62:428–37.

Dimpfel, W., Spuler, M., Pierau, F.K., Thioctic acid induces dose-dependent sprouting of neurites in cultured rat neuroblastoma cells. Developmental Pharmacology and Therapeutics (1990).14: 193–99.

Doelman, C.J., Bast, A., Oxygen radicals in lung pathology. Department of Pharmacochemistry, Faculty of Chemistry Vrije Universiteit, Amsterdam, The Netherlands. Free Radic Biol Med 1990;9(5):381–400.

Dorofeeva, G., Bondar, L., Lepikhov, P., Prilutskii, A., Characteristics of the functional state of the pancreas, lipid peroxidation and antioxidant defense in food hypersensitivity in children. Pediatriia 1992;(3):18–22.

Evans D.A., Morris, M.C., Is a randomized trial of antioxidants in the primary prevention of Alzheimer's disease warranted? Rush Alzheimer's Disease Center, Rush University, Chicago. Alzheimer Dis Assoc Disord 1996 Fall;10 Suppl 1:45–9.

Famulari, A.L., Sacerdote de Lustig, E., Reides, C., The antioxidant enzymatic blood profile in Alzheimer's and vascular diseases. Their association and a possible assay to differentiate demented subjects and controls. Hospital Sirio-Libanes, FACENE, Buenos Aires, Argentina. J Neurol Sci 1996 Sep 15;141(1–2):69–78.

Faust, A., Burkart, V., Ulrich, H., Weischer, C., Kolb, H. Effect of Alpha Lipoic Acid on cyclophosphamide-induced diabetes and insulitis in non-obese diabetic mice. Diabetes Research Institute, University of Düsseldorf, Germany. Int J Immunopharmacol 1994 Jan;16(1):61–66.

Flannery, G., Burroughs, A., Butler, P., Chelliah, J., Hamilton-Miller J,, Brumfitt, W., Baum, H. Antimitochondrial antibodies in primary biliary cirrhosis recognize both specific peptides and shared epitopes of the M2 family of antigens. Hepatology 1989 Sep;10(3):370–74.

Freed, B., Rapoport. et al., Inhibition of early events in the human T-lymphocyte response to mitogens and allo-gantigens by hydrogen peroxide. Arch Surg (1987) 122: 99–104.

Fregeau, D., Roche, T., Davis, P., Coppel R., Gershwin M., J Immunol 1990 Mar 1;144(5):1671+.

Fujiwara, K., Okamura-Ikeda, K., Motokawa, Y., Assay for protein lipoylation reaction. Institute for Enzyme Research, University of Tokushima, Japan. Methods Enzymol 1995;251:340–47.

Fujiwara, K., Okamura-Ikeda, K., Motokawa, Y., cDNA sequence, in vitro synthesis, and intramitochondrial lipoylation of H-protein of the glycine cleavage system. J Biol Chem 1990 Oct 15;265(29):17463–67.

Fujiwara, K., Okamura-Ikeda, K, Motokawa, Y., Lipoylation of H-protein of the glycine cleavage system. The effect of site-directed metagenesis of amino acid residues around the lipoyllysine residue on the lipoic acid attachment.

Fussey, S., Bassendine, M., James, O., Yeaman, S., Characterisation of the reactivity of autoantibodies in primary biliary cirrhosis. Biochem Biophys Res Commun 1989 Jul 31;162(2):658–63.

Garganta, C.L., Wolf, B., Lipoamidase activity in human serum is due to biotinidase. Clin Chim Acta 1990 Aug 31;189(3):313–25.

Ghadge, G.D., Lee, J.P., Bindokas, V.P., Jordan, J., Ma, L., Miller, R.J., Roos, R.P., Mutant superoxide dismutase-1-linked familial amyotrophic lateral sclerosis: molecular mechanisms of neuronal death and protection. Department of Neurology, The University of Chicago, Chicago, Illinois 60637, USA. J Neurosci 1997 Nov 15;17(22):8756–66.

Gotz, M.E., Dirr, A., Gsell, W., Burger, R., Janetzky, B., Freyberger, A., Reichmann, H., Rausch, W.D., Riederer, P., Influence of N-methyl-4-phenyl-1,2,3,6-tetrahydropyridine, Alpha Lipoic Acid and L-deprenyl on the interplay between cellular redox systems. J Neural Transm Suppl 1994;43:145–62.

Gregus, Z., Stein, Varga, Effect of Alpha Lipoic Acid on biliary excretion of glutathione and metals. Toxicol Appl Pharmcol (1992)114: 86–96.

Gries, F.A., Ziegler, D., Hanefeld, M., Rulinau, K.J., Meipner, H.B., Symtomatic diabetic peripheral ItA4 neuropathy With the anti-oxidant alpha -Lipoic Acid: A 3-week multicentre randomized controlled trial. *Oxidants and Antioxidants in Biology,* Oxygen Club of California, Annual Meeting, March 1995.

Gut, J., Christen, U., Frey, N., Koch, V., Stoffler, D., Molecular mimicry in halothane hepatitis: biochemical and structural characterization of lipoylated autoantigens. Toxicology 1995 Mar 31;97(1–3):199–224.

Han, D., Handelman, G.J., Packer, L., Analysis of reduced and oxidized Alpha Lipoic Acid in biological samples by high-performance liquid chromatography. Methods Enzymol 1995;251:315–25.

Han, D., Packer, L., A-Lipoic Acid Modulation of Glutathione in a Human T-lymphocyte cell line. *Oxidants and Antioxidants in Biology,* Oxygen Club of California, Annual Meeting, March 1995.

Han, D., Tritschler, H.J., Packer, L., Alpha Lipoic Acid increases intracellular glutathione in a human T-lymphocyte Jurkat cell line. Biochem Biophys Res Commun 1995 Feb 6;207(1):258–64.

Haramaki, N., Assadnazari, H., Zimmer, G., Schepkin, V., Packer, L., The influence of vitamin E and dihydrolipoic acid on cardiac energy and gluththione status under hypoxia-reoxygenation. Department of Molecular and Cell Biology, University of California, Berkeley Biochem Mol Biol Int 1995 Oct;37(3):591–97.

Haramaki, N., Packer, L., et al. Cardiac recovery during post-ischemic reperfusion is improved by combination of vitamin E with dihydrolipoic acid. Biochemical and Biophysical Research (1993). Vol 196, No. 3, 1101–7. [b]

Harding, J.J., Cigarettes and cataract: cadmium or a lack of Vitamin C? [editorial; comment]. Br J Ophthalmol 1995 Mar;79(3):199–200.

Harmon, D., Free radical involvement in aging: pathophysiology and therapeutic implications. Drugs Aging 3: 1993, 60–80.

Hatch, G.E., Asthma, inhaled oxidants, and dietary antioxidants. Pulmonary Toxicology Branch, U.S. Environmental Protection Agency, Research Triangle Park, NC, Am J Clin Nutr 1995 Mar;61(3 Suppl):625S–30S.

Haugaard, N., Stimulation of glucose utilization by thioctic acid in rat diaphragm incubated in vitro. Biochemica et Biophysica ACTA (1970). 583–86.

Heliovaara, M., Knekt, P., Aho, K., Aaran, R.K., Alfthan, G., Aromaa A Serum antioxidants and risk of rheumatoid arthritis. Social Insurance Institution, Helsinki, Finland. Ann Rheum Dis 1994 Jan;53(1):51–53.

Henriksen, E.J., Jacob, S., Streeper, R.S., Fogt, D.L., Hokama, J.Y., Tritschler, H.J., Stimulation by alpha-lipoic acid of glucose transport activity in skeletal muscle of lean and obese Zucker rats. Department of Physiology, University of Arizona, Tucson Life Sci 1997;61(8):805–12.

Henrotin, Y., Deby-Dupont, G., Deby, C., Franchimont, P., Emerit, I., Active oxygen species, articular inflammation and cartilage damage. University Sart-Tilman, Liege, Belgium. EXS 1992 62:308–22.

Hofmann, M., Mainka, P., Tritschler, H., Fuchs, J., Decrease of red cell membrane fluidity and -SH groups due to hyperglycemic conditions is counteracted by Alpha Lipoic Acid. Arch Biochem Biophys 1995 Dec 1;324 (1): 85–92.

Honkanen, V., The factors affecting plasma glutathione peroxidase and selenium in rheumatoid arthritis: a multiple linear regression analysis. Scand J Rheumatol 1991;20(6):385–91.

Jacob, S., Henriksen, E., Schiemann, A., Simon, I, Clancy, D.E., Tritschler, H.J., Jung, W.I., Enhancement of glucose disposal in patients with type 2 diabetes by Alpha Lipoic Acid. Arzneimittelforschung 1995 Aug;45(8):872–74.

Jacob, S., Henriksen, E.J., Tritschler, H.J., Augustin, H.J., Dietze, G.J., Improvement of insulin-stimulated glucose-disposal in type 2 diabetes after repeated parenteral administration of thioctic acid. Hypertension and Diabetes Research Unit, Max Grundig Clinic, Buhl, Germany. Exp Clin Endocrinol Diabetes 1996;104(3):284–88. [b]

Jacob, S., Streeper, R.S., Fogt, D.L., Hokama, J.Y., Tritschler, H.J., Dietze, G.J., Henriksen, E.J., The antioxidant alpha-lipoic acid enhances insulin-stimulated glucose metabolism in insulin-resistant rat skeletal muscle. Department of Physiology, University of Arizona College of Medicine, Tucson. Diabetes 1996 Aug;45(8):1024–29.

Jacques, P., et al., Long-term vitamin C supplement use and prevalence of early age-related opacities. American Journal of Clinical Nutrition, 1997, 66: 911–16.

Jayanthi, S., Jayanthi, G., Varalakshmi, P., Effect of DL Alpha Lipoic Acid on some carbohydrate metabolizing enzymes in stone forming rats. Department of Medical Biochemistry, University of Madras, India Biochem Int 1991 Sep;25(1):123–36.

Jayanthi, S., Saravanan, N., Varalakshmi, P., Effect of DL Alpha Lipoic Acid in glyoxylate-induced acute lithiasis. Department of Medical Biochemistry, Dr A.L. Mudaliar Post Graduate Institute of Basic Medical Sciences, University of Madras, India. Pharmacol Res 1994 Oct–Nov;30 (3):281–88.

Jayanthi, S., Varalakshmi, P., Tissue lipids in experimental calcium oxalate lithiasis and the effect of DL Alpha Lipoic Acid. Department of Medical Biochemistry, Dr. A.L.M. P.G.I.B.M.S, University of Madras, India. Biochem Int 1992 Apr;26(5):913–21.

Jorg, J., Metz, F., Scharafinski, H., "Drug treatment of diabetic polyneuropathy with Alpha Lipoic Acid or Vitamin B preparations. A clinical and neurophysiologic study. Neurologische Universitatskliniken Lubeck und Essen. Nervenarzt 1988 Jan;59(1):36–44.

Julius, M., et al., Glutathione and Mordidity in a Community-based sample of elderly. Journal of Clinical Epidemiology. 47:9(1994), 1021–26.

Junqueira,V., Barros, A.P., Fuzaro, T., da Silva, S., Chan, V., et al., Decreasing blood oxidative stress status in coronary heart disease patients by oral antioxidant supplementation. *Oxidants and Antioxidants in Biology*, Oxygen Club of California, Annual Meeting, March 1995.

Kagan, V., Freisleben, H., Tsuchiya, M., Forte, T., Packer, L., "Generation of probucol radicals and their reduction by ascorbate and dihydroAlpha Lipoic Acid in human low density lipoproteins. Department of Molecular and Cell Biology, University of California, Berkeley 94720. Free Radic Res Commun 1991; 15(5): 265–76. [a]

Kagan, V., Serbinova, E., Forte, T., Scita, G., Packer, L., Recycling of vitamin E in human low density lipoproteins. J Lipid Res 1992 Mar;33(3):385–97.

Kagan, V., Shvedova, A., Serbinova, E., Dihydrolipoic acid—a universal antioxidant both in the membrane and in the aqueous phase. Reduction of peroxyl, ascorbyl and chromanoxyl radicals. Department of Molecular and Cell Biology, University of California, Berkeley 94270. Biochem Pharmacol 1992 Oct 20;44(8): 1637–49.

Kagan, V., Yalowich, J., Day, B., Goldman, R., Gantchev, T., Stoyanovsky, D., Ascorbate is the primary reductant of the phenoxyl radical of etoposide in the presence of thiols both in cell homogenates and in model systems. Department of Environmental and Occupational Health, University of Pittsburgh, Pennsylvania 15238. Biochemistry 1994 Aug 16;33(32):9651–60.

Kahler, W., Kuklinski, B., Ruhlmann, C., Plotz, C., Diabetes mellitus—a free radical-associated disease. Results of adjuvant antioxidant supplementation] Klinik fur Innere Medizin, Klinikums Rostock-Sudstadt. Z Gesamte Inn Med 1993 May;48(5):223–32.

Kawabata, T., Packer, L., Alpha-lipoic acid can protect against glycation of serum albumin, but not low density lipoprotein. Biochem Biophys Res Commun 1994 Aug 30;203(1):99–104.

Keith, R.L., Setiarahardjo, I., Fernando, Q., Aposhian, H.V., Gandolfi, A., Utilization of renal slices to evaluate the efficacy of chelating agents for removing mercury from the kidney. Center for Toxicology, University of Arizona, Tucson. Toxicology 1997 Jan 15;116(1–3):67–75.

Kilic, F., Handelman, G.J., Serbinova, E., Packer, L., Trevithick, J.R., Modelling cortical cataractogenesis 17: in vitro effect of a-Alpha Lipoic Acid on glucose-induced lens membrane damage, a model of diabetic cataractogenesis. Dept. of Biochemistry, University of Western Ontario, London, Canada. Biochem Mol Biol Int 1995 Oct;37(2):361–70.

Kilic, F., Packer. L., Trevethick, J.R., Modeling corticol cataractogenesis 17: In vitro effect of a-Alpha Lipoic Acid on glucose-induced lens membrane damage, a model of diabetic cataractogenesis. Exp Eye Res (1994). [b]

Kis, K., Meier, T., Multhoff, G., Issels, R., Lipoic acid modulation of lymphocyte cysteine uptake. Institute for Klinische Hamatologie, GSF Forschungszentrum for Umwelt and Gesundeit.

Klein, B.E., Klein, R., Linton, K.L., Franke, T., Cigarette smoking and lens opacities. The Beaver Dam Eye Study Department of Ophthalmology, University of Wisconsin, Madison. Am J Prev Med 1993 Jan–Feb;9(1):27–30, Comment in: Am J Prev Med 1993 Jan–Feb;9(1):65–66.

Komeshima, N., Osawa, T., Nishitoba, T., Jinno, Y., Kiriu, T., Synthesis and anti-inflammatory activity of antioxidants, 4-alkylthio-o-anisidine derivatives. Pharmaceutical Research

Laboratory, Kirin Brewery Co., Ltd., Gunma, Japan. Chem Pharm Bull (Tokyo) 1992 Feb;40(2):351–66.

Korkina, L.G., Afanasef, I.B., et al., Antioxidant therapy in children affected by irradiation from the Chernobyl nuclear accident. Biochem Soc Trans (1993) 21: 314S.

Kropachova, K., Mishurova, E., Flavobion and thioctacid lessen irradiation-induced latent injury of the liver, Biull Eksp Biol Med 1992 May;113(5):547–49.

Lahoda, F., Therapeutic possibilities in polyneuropathies. Fortschr Med 1982 Oct 14;100(38):1759–60.

Lang, et al., Low blood glutathione levels in healthy aging adults, Journal of Laboratory and Clinical Medicine, 120:5 (1992) 720–25.

Legrand-Poels, S., Vaira, D., et al., Activation of human immunodeficiency virus type 1 by oxidative stress. AIDS Res Human Retrovir (1990) 6:1389–97.

Leung, P.S., Iwayama, T., Coppel, R.L., Gershwin, M.E., Site-directed metagenesis of lysine within the immunodominant autoepitope of PDC-E2. Division of Rheumatology, Allergy and Clinical Immunology, University of California, Davis. Hepatology 1990 Dec;12(6):1321–28.

Lin, R.C., Antony, V., Lumeng L., Li, T.K., Mai, K., Liu, C., Wang, Q.D., et al. Alcohol Clin Exp Res 1994 Dec;18(6): 1443-47.

Loffelhardt, S., Bonaventura, C., Locher, M., Borbe, H.O., Bisswanger, H., Interaction of Alpha Lipoic Acid enantiomers and homologues with the enzyme components of the mammalian pyruvate dehydrogenase complex. Biochem Pharmacol 1995 Aug 25;50(5):637–46.

Low, P.A., Nickander, K., Schmelzer, L.D., Kihara, M., Nagamatsu M., Tritschler, H., Experimental diabetic neuropathy: idcremia, oxidative stress, and neuroprotection. Mayo Foundation and Asta Medica Dresden, Germany, *Oxidants and Antioxidants in Biology,* Oxygen Club of California, Annual Meeting, March 1995.

Maarten C., et al., Dietary antioxidants in Parkinson's disease: The Rotterdam study. Archives of Neurology 1997, 54(6):762–65.

Maitra, I., Serbinova, E., Trischler, H., Packer, L., Alpha Lipoic Acid prevents buthionine sulfoximine-induced cataract formation in newborn rats. Free Radic Biol Med 1995 Apr;18(4):823–29.

Mares-Perlman, J.A., Brady, W.E., Klein, R., Klein, B.E., Bowen, P., Stacewicz-Sapuntzakis, M., Palta, M., Serum antioxidants and age-related macular degeneration in a population-based case-control study. Arch Ophthalmol 1995 Dec;113(12): 1518–23.

Matsugo, S., Yan, L.J., Han, D., Trischler, H.J., Packer, L. Elucidation of antioxidant activity of alpha lipoic acid toward hydroxyl radical. Biochem Biophys Res Commun 1995 Mar 8;208(1):161–67.

McAlindon, T.E., Jacques, P., Zhang, Y., et. al., Do antioxidant micronutrients protect against the development and progression of knee osteoarthritis? Arthritis Center, Boston U Med Cen, Arthritis Rheum 1996 Apr;39(4):648–56.

McCarty, M.F., Rubin, E.J., Rationales for micronutrient supplementation in diabetes. Med Hypotheses 1984 Feb;13(2):139-51.

Messent, M., Sinclair, D.G., Quinlan, G.J., Mumby, S.E., Gutteridge, J.M., Evans, T.W., Pulmonary vascular permeability after cardiopulmonary bypass and its relationship to oxidative stress. Unit of Critical Care, National Heart and Lung Institute, London, UK. Crit Care Med 1997 Mar;25(3):425–29.

Meydani, S., et al., Vitamin E supplementation and in vivo immune response in healthy elderly subjects. Journal of the American Medical Association. 1997, 277(17):1333–416.

Michiels, C., Arnould, T., Thibaut-Vercruyssen, R., Bouaziz, N., Perfused human saphenous veins for the study of the origin of varicose veins: role of the endothelium and of hypoxia. Laboratoire de Biochimie Cellulaire, Facultes

Universitaires, Notre Dame de l Paix, Namur, Belgium. Int Angiol 1997 Jun;16(2):134–41.

Mizuno, M., Packer, L., Suppression of protooncogene c-fos expression by antioxidant dihydroAlpha Lipoic Acid. Department of Molecular and Cell Biology, University of California, Berkeley. Methods Enzymol 1995;252:180–86.

Morgan, M.Y., Hepatoprotective agents in alcoholic liver disease. Acta Med Scand Suppl 1985;703:225–33.

Morris, C.J., Earl, J.R., Trenam, C.W., Blake, D.R., Reactive oxygen species and iron—a dangerous partnership in inflammation. Int J Biochem Cell Biol 1995 Feb;27(2):109–22.

Muller, L., Synergistic effects of alpha-tocopherol and Alpha Lipoic Acid on reactive oxygen species in blood, Institute of Toxicology, University of Düssseldorf, FRG. Toxicology 1989 Oct 2; 58(2):175–85.

Muller, L., Menzel, H.T.I., Studies on the efficacy of lipoic acid and dihydrolipoate in the alteration of cadmium2+ toxicity in isolated hepatocytes. Biochim Biophys Acta 1990 May 22;1052(3):386–91. [b]

Nagamatsu, M., Nickander, K.K., Schmelzer, J.D., Raya, A., Wittrock, D.A., Tritschler, H., Low, P.A., "Lipoic Acid improves nerve blood flow, reduces oxidative stress, and improves distal nerve conduction in experimental diabetic neuropathy." Diabetes Care 1995 Aug;18(8):1160–67.

Nilsson, L., Ronge, E., Lipoamidase and biotinidase deficiency: evidence that lipoamidase and biotinidase are the same enzyme in human serum. Eur J Clin Chem Clin Biochem 1992 Mar;30(3):119–26.

Novak, Z., Nemeth, I., Gyurkovits, K., Varga, S.I., Matkovics, B., Examination of the role of oxygen free radicals in bronchial asthma in childhood. Clin Chim Acta 1991 Sep 30;201(3):247–51.

Offen, D., Ziv, I., Sternin, H., Melamed, E., Hochman, A., Prevention of dopamine-induced cell death by thiol antioxidants: possible implications for treatment of Parkinson's disease. Department of Neurology, Beilinson Medical Center, Petah-Tiqva, Israel. Exp Neurol 1996 Sep;141(1): 32–39.

Olin, K.L., Morse, L.S., Murphy, C., Paul-Murphy, J., Line, S., Bellhorn, R.W., Hjelmeland, L.M., Keen, C.L., Trace element status and free radical defense in elderly rhesus macaques (Macaca mulatta) with macular drusen. University of California, Davis 95616. Proc Soc Exp Biol Med 1995 Apr;208(4):370–77.

Oka, Y., Arakawa, S., Kamidono, S., Saito, S.A., Study of middle-high aged impotent patients. Department of Urology, Kobe University, School of Medicine. Nippon Hinyokika Gakkai Zasshi 1995 Aug;86(8):1336–45.

O'Neill, C.A., Halliwell, B., van der Vliet, A., Davis, P.A., Packer, L., Tritschler, H., Strohman, W.J., Rieland, T, Cross, C.E., Reznick, A.Z., Aldehyde-induced protein modifications in human plasma: protection by glutathione and dihydroAlpha Lipoic Acid. J Lab Clin Med 1994 Sep;124(3):359–70.

Ou, P., Nourooz-Zadeh, J., Tritschler, H.J., Wolff, S.P., Activation of aldose reductase in rat lens and metal-ion chelation by aldose reductase inhibitors and lipoic acid. Department of Medicine, University College London, England. SOURCE: Free Radic Res 1996 Oct;25(4):337–46.

Ou, P., Tritschler, H.J., Wolff, S.P., Thioctic (lipoic) acid: a therapeutic metal-chelating antioxidant? Department of Medicine, University College London Medical School, U.K. Biochem Pharmacol 1995 Jun 29;50(1):123–26. [b]

Packer, L., Antioxidant properties of Alpha Lipoic Acid and its therapeutic effects in prevention of diabetes complications and cataracts. Ann N Y Acad Sci 1994 Nov 17;738: 257–64. [a]

Packer, L., New horizons in antioxidant research: action of thioctic acid/dihydrolipic acid couple in biological systems, 35–45.

Packer, L., "New horizons in vitamin E research—the vitamin E cycle, biochemistry, and clinical applications Lipid-Soluble Antioxidants: Biochemistry and Clinical Applications (1992).

Packer, L., "Protective role of vitamin E in biological systems. Department of Molecular and Cell Biology, University of California, Berkeley. Am J Clin Nutr 1991 Apr;53(4 Suppl):1050S–55S.

Packer, L., Suzuki, "Vitamin E and alpha lipoic acid: role in antioxidant recycling and activation of the NF-KB transcription factor. Molec Aspects Med (1993). [e]

Packer, L., Witt, E.H., Tritschler, H.J. Alph Lipoic Acid as a biological antioxidant. Free Radic Biol Med 1995 Aug;19(2):227–50.

Panigrahi, M., Sadguna, Y., et al. Alpha lipid acid protects against reperfusion injury following cerebral ischemia in rats. Department of Neurochemistry, National Institue of Mental Health and Neurosciences, Bangalore, India. Brain Research 1996 Apr 22; 717(1–2):184–8.

Parish, R.C., Doering P.L., Treatment of Amanita mushroom poisoning: a review. Vet Hum Toxicol 1986 Aug;28(4):318–22.

Patel, M.S., Vettakkorumakankav, N.N., Liu, T.C., Dihydrolipoamide dehydrogenase: activity assays. Methods Enzymol 1995;252:186–95.

Paydas, S., Kocak, R., Erturk, F., Erken, E., Zaksu, H.S., Gurcay, A., Poisoning due to amatoxin-containing Lepiota species. Department of Internal Medicine, Cukurova University Medical School, Adana, Turkey. Br J Clin Pract 1990 Nov;44(11):450–53.

Pick, U., Haramaki, N., Constantinescu, A., Handelman, G.J, Tritschler, H.J., Packer, L., Glutathione reductase and lipoamide dehydrogenase have opposite stereospecificities for Alpha Lipoic Acid enantiomers. Biochem Biophys Res Commun 1995 Jan 17;206(2):724–30.

Piering, W.F., Bratanow, N., Role of the clinical laboratory in guiding treatment of Amanita virosa mushroom poisoning: report of two cases. Clin Chem 1990 Mar;36 (3):571–74.

Podda, M., Koh, B., Descans, B., Rallis, M., Packer L., Penetration, reduction, and protective effects if alpha lipoic acid in UV–exposed skin, *Oxidants and Antioxidants in Biology,* Oxygen Club of California, Annual Meeting, March 1995. [a]

Podda, M., Tritschler, H.J., Ulrich, H., Packer, L. Alpha lipoic acid supplementation prevents symptoms of vitamin E deficiency." Department of Molecular and Cell Biology, University of California at Berkeley, 94720-3200. Biochem Biophys Res Commun 1994 Oct 14;204(1):98–104.

Powell, C.V., Nash, A.A., Powers, H.J., Primhak, R.A., Antioxidant status in asthma. Children's Hospital, Western Bank, Sheffield, United Kingdom. Pediatr Pulmonol 1994 Jul;18(1):34–38.

Ramakrishnan, S., Wolfe, Catravas., Radioprotection of hematopic tissues in mice by alpha lipoic acid. Radiation Research (1992) 130:360–65.

Ramakrishnan, S., Sulochana, K.N., Selvaraj, T., Abdul Rahim A., Lakshmi M., Arunagiri, K., Smoking of beedies and cataract: cadmium and vitamin C in the lens and blood. Medical and Vision Research Foundations, Madras, India. Br J Ophthalmol 1995 Mar;79(3):202–26.

Remacle, J., Arnould, T., Michiels, C., The relation between venous stasis and the occurrence of pain. Laboratoire de Biochimie Cellulaire, Facultés Universitaires Notre-Dame de la Paix, Bruxelles, Belgique. Phlebologie 1992 Jan–Mar;45(1):33–37; discussion 38–39.

Ron, G.I., Shmeleva, L.T., Klein, A.V., Iashkova, E., Lipid peroxidation and the status of the basal membrane of the acinar cells in the minor salivary glands of patients with Sjögren's syndrome. Stomatologiia (Mosk) 1992 Mar–Apr; (2):23–26.

Rosenberg, H., Culik, R., Effect of DL alpha lipoic acid in glyoxylate-induced acute lithiasis. The Italian Pharmacological Society (1994) Vol. 80, 86–90.

Rucker, R.B., Wold, F., Cofactors in and as posttranslational protein modifications. FASEB J 1988 Apr;2(7):2252–61.

Sachse, G., Willms, B. Efficacy of thioctic acid in the therapy of peripheral diabetic neuropathy. Horm Metab Res Suppl 1980; 9:105–7.

Said, H.M., Redha, R., Nylander, W.A. Carrier-mediated, Na+ gradient-dependent transport for biotin in human intestinal brush-border membrane vesicles.Vanderbilt University School of Medicine, Am J Physiol 1987 Nov; 253 (5 Pt 1):G631–36.

Sandhya, P. Effect of lipoic acid administration on gentamicin-induced lipid peroxidation in rats. Department of Medical Biochemistry, Post Graduate Institute of Basic Medical Sciences, University of Madras, Taramani Campus, India. J Appl Toxicol 1997 Nov–Dec;17(6):405–8.

Sano, M., et al. A controlled trial of selegiline, alpha-tocopherol, or both as treatment for Alzheimer's disease, New England Journal of Medicine 1997 336(17).

Scheer, B., Zimmer, G. DHLA prevents hypoxic/reoxygenation and peroxidative damage in rat heart mitochondria. Arch Biochem Biophys (1993) 302:385–90.

Schepkin, V., Kawabata. T., Packer, L., NMR study of alpha lipoic acid binding to bovine serum albumin. Biochem Mol Biol Int 1994 Aug;33(5):879–86.

Schmidt, R., Fazekas, F., Hayn, M., Schmidt, H., Kapeller, P., Roob, G., Offenbacher, H., Schumacher, M., et al., Risk factors for microangiopathy-related cerebral damage in the Austrian stroke prevention study. Department of Neurology, Karl-Franzens University Graz, Austria. SOURCE: J Neurol Sci 1997 Nov 6;152(1):15–21.

Seaton, T.A., Jenner, P., A report on the effects of acute and subacute administration of R- and 5-thioctic acid on 14 C-deoxyglucose utilization in rat brain (1992).

Seddon, J.M., Ajani, U.A., Sperduto. R.D., Hiller, R., Blair, N., Burton, T.C., Farber, M.D., Gragoudas, E.S., Haller, J., et al., Dietary carotenoids, vitamins A, C, and E, and advanced age-related macular degeneration. Eye Disease Case-Control Study Group [see comments] [published erratum appears in JAMA 1995 Feb 22;273(8):622] JAMA 1994 Nov 9;272(18):1413–20.

Serbinova, E., Shamsuddin, K., et al., Thioctic acid protects against ischemia-reperfusion injury in the isolated perfused langendorf heart. Free Rad Res Comms (1992) Vol 17:1, 49–58.

Shalini, V.K., Luthra, M., Srinivas, L., Rao, S.H., Basti, S., Reddy, M., Balasubramanian, D., Oxidative damage to the eye lens caused by cigarette smoke and fuel smoke condensates. Centre for Cellular and Molecular Biology, Hyderabad, India. Indian J Biochem Biophys 1994 Aug; 31(4):261–66.

Shvedova, A.A., Kisin, E.R., Kagan, V.E., Karol, M.H., Increased lipid peroxidation and decreased antioxidants in lungs of guinea pigs following an allergic pulmonary response. Toxicol Appl Pharmacol 1995 May;132(1): 72–81.

Shoji, S., Furuishi, K., Misumi, S., Miyazaki, T., Kino, M., Yamataka, K., Thiamine disulfide as a potent inhibitor of human immunodeficiency virus (type-1) production. Biochem Biophys Res Commun 1994 Nov 30;205(1):967–75.

Smith, L.J., Houston, M., Anderson, J. Increased levels of glutathione in bronchoalveolar lavage fluid from patients with asthma. Am Rev Respir Dis 1993 Jun;147(6 Pt 1):1461–64.

Snodderly, D.M. Evidence for protection against age-related macular degeneration by carotenoids and antioxidant vitamins. Schepens Eye Research Institute, Macular

Disease Research Center, Am J Clin Nutr 1995 Dec;62 (6 Suppl):1448S–61S.

Sopher, B.L., Martin, G.M., Furlong, C.E., Kavanagh, T.J., Fukuchi, K., Neurodegenerative mechanisms in Alzheimer's disease. A role for oxidative damage in amyloid beta protein precursor-mediated cell death. Mol Chem Neuropathol 1996 Oct–Dec;29(2–3):153–68.

Stoll, S., Hartmann, H., et al., The potent free radical scavenger alpha lipoic acid improved memory in aged mice. Putative relationship to NMDA receptor deficits. Pharmacol Biochem Behav (1993) 36:799–805.

Strodter, D., Lehmann, E., Lehmann, U., Tritschler, H.J., Bretzel R.G., Federlin K., The influence of thioctic acid on metabolism and function of the diabetic heart. Medical Clinic III, University of Giessen, Germany. Diabetes Res Clin Pract 1995 Jul;29(1):19–26.

Studt, J., Heuer, L.J., Diabetic autonomic neuropathy of the heart and its treatment with thioctic acid. Dtsch Z Verdau Stoffwechselkr 1984;44(4): 173–80.

Sumathi, R., Jayanthi, S., Kalpanadevi, V., Varalakshmi, P., Effect of DL alpha lipoic acid on tissue lipid peroxidation and antioxidant systems in normal and glycollate treated rats. Pharmacol Res 1993 May–Jun;27(4): 309–18. [a]

Sumathi, R., Devi, Varalakshmi, D., L alpha lipoic acid protection against cadmium-induced tissue peroxidation. Med Sci Res (1994) 22: 23–25. [b]

Suzuki., Y.J., Mizuno, M., Tritschler, H.J., Packer, L., "Regulation of NF-kappa-B DNA binding activity by dihydrolipoate. Department of Molecular and Cell Biology, Biochem Mol Biol Int 1995 Jun;36(2):241–46. [a]

Suzuki, Y.J., Tsuchiya, M., Packer, L., Lipoic acid prevents glucose-induced protein modifications. Department of Molecular and Cell Biology, University of California, Berkeley. Free Radic Res Commun 1992;17(3):211–17. [b]

Suzuki, Y.J., Tsuchiya, M., Packer, L., Thiotic acid and dihydrolipoic acid are novel antioxidants which interact with reactive oxygen species. Free Rad Res Comm (1991), 15: (5):255–63. [c]

Spoerke, D.G., Smolinske, S.C., Wruk, K.M., Rumack, B.H., Infrequently used antidotes: indications and availability. Vet Hum Toxicol 1986 Feb;28(1):69–75.

Teichert, J., Preiss, R.H., PLC-methods for determination of alpha lipoic acid and its reduced form in human plasma. Institute of Clinical Pharmacology, University of Leipzig, Germany. Biochem Biophys Res Commun 1992 Dec 30; 189 (3):1709–15. [a]

Teichert, J., Preiss, R. Determination of alpha lipoic acid in human plasma by high-performance liquid chromatography with electrochemical detection. J Chromatogr B Biomed Appl 1995 Oct 20;672(2):277–81. [b]

Trevino, R.J., Air pollution and its effect on the upper respiratory tract and on allergic rhinosinusitis. Otolaryngol Head Neck Surg 1996 Feb;114(2): 239–41.

Trevithick, J.R., Kilic, F., Handelman, G.J., Serbinow E., Packer, L., In vitro effect of alpha lipoic acid on glucose-induced lens membrane damage, a model of diabetic cataractgenesis. University of Western Ontario, London, Ontario, and University of California, Berkeley, *Oxidants and Antioxidants in Biology,* Oxygen Club of California, Annual Meeting, March 1995.

Tritschler, H.J., Wolff, S.P., Thioctic (lipoic) acid: a therapeutic metal-chelating antioxidant? Biochem Pharmacol 1995 Jun 29;50(1):123–26.

Troisi, R.J., Willett, W.C., Weiss, S.T., Trichopoulos, D., Rosner, B., Speizer F.E., A prospective study of diet and adult-onset asthma [see comments]. Am J Respir Crit Care Med 1995 May;151(5):1401–8 Comment in: Am J Respir Crit Care Med 1995 May;151(5):1292–93.

Tsuchiya, Thompson, Suzuki, et. al., Superoxide formed from cigarette smoke impairs polymorphononuclear leukocyte active oxygen generation activity. Arch Biochem Biophys (1992) 299: 30–37.

Vaage, J., Antonelli M., Bufi M., Irtun O., DeBlasi R.A., Corbucci G.G., Gasparetto A., Semb, A.G., Exogenous reactive oxygen species deplete the isolated rat heart of antioxidants. Department of Surgery, University of Tromso, Norway. Free Radic Biol Med 1997;22(1–2):85–92.

Van der Vliet, A., Cross, C.E., Halliwell, B., O'Neill, C., Plasma protein sulfhydryl oxidation: effect of low molecular weight thiols. Department of Internal Medicine, UCD Medical Center, U of C, Sacramento Methods Enzymol 1995;251:448–55.

Walter, M.F., Mason, R.P., Mason, P.E., Alzheimer's disease amyloid beta peptide 25-35 inhibits lipid eroxidation as a result of its membrane interactions. Laboratory for Membrane Structure Studies, MCP-Hahnemann School of Medicine, Allegheny University of the Health Sciences, Pittsburgh, PA, Biochem Biophys Res Commun 1997 Apr 28;233(3):760–64.

West, S., Munoz, B., Schein, O.D., Vitale, S., Maguire, M., Taylor, H.R., Bressler, N.M., Cigarette smoking and risk for progression of nuclear opacities. Dana Center for Preventive Opthalmology, Wilmer Institute, Johns Hopkins University, Baltimore, MD, Arch Ophthalmol 1995 Nov;113(11):1377–80.

Whiteman, M., Tritschler, H., Halliwell, B., Protection against peroxynitrite-dependent tyrosine nitration and alpha 1-antiproteinase inactivation by oxidized and reduced Alpha Lipoic Acid. Neurodegenerative Disease Research Centre, King's College, London, UK. FEBS Lett 1996 Jan 22;379(1):74–76.

Wickramasinghe, S.N., Hasan, R., In vitro effects of vitamin C, thioctic acid and dihydro Alpha Lipoic Acid on the cytotoxicity of post-ethanol serum. Dept. of Haematology, St. Mary's Hospital Medical School, Imperial College of Science, London, U.K. Biochem Pharmacol 1992 Feb 4;43(3):407–11.

Yan, Liang-Jun, Packer, L., Alpha lipoic acid protects apolo-proteins B-100 of human low density liproteins against oxidative modifications mediated by hypochlorite. *Oxidants and Antioxidants in Biology*, Oxygen Club of California, Annual Meeting, March 1995.

Yoshida, I., Sweetman, L., Kulovich, S., Nyhan, W.L., Rob-inson, B.H., Effect of Alpha Lipoic Acid in a patient with defective activity of pyruvate dehydrogenase, 2-oxoglutar-ate dehydrogenase, and branched-chain keto acid dehydro-genase. Kurume University, Japan. Pediatr Res 1990 Jan;27(1):75–79.

Yuichiro, J., Suzuki, Masahiki, Thioctic acid and dihydroli-poic acid are novel antioxidants which interact with reac-tive oxygen species. Free Radical Research Comms (1991) Vol. 15:No. 5, 255–63.

Zhang, Hwang, Sevanian, Dwyer, Dependence of the LDL oxidative susceptibility on the LDL cholesterol protein ratio and a-tocopherol content in human plasma. *Oxidants and Antioxidants in Biology*, Oxygen Club of California, Annual Meeting, March 1995.

Ziegler, D., Conrad, F., Ulrich, H. et. al., Effects of treat-ment with the antioxidant alpha lipoic acid on cardiac autonomic neuropathy in NIDDM patients—a 4-month ran-domized controlled multicenter—trial (DEKAN Study).

Note: Many of the studies discussed in this book are animal studies. While not all data in animal studies can be applied 100% to humans for a number of reasons, they are of great scientific value.

Animals are valuable experimental tools because they do not respond to the placebo effect, which otherwise can greatly distort human research results. In humans, the average placebo response is over 60%, and may be as high as 100%. This, of course, is one of the reasons that a good valid human study should be double-blind, cross-over in design.

As scientists we understand that there is a need to use laboratory animals for the purposes of education; as human beings we can only hope that all animals used for testing purposes were treated as humanely as possible.

Dr. Beth M. Ley Jacobs

Beth M. Ley Jacobs, Ph.D., has been a science writer specializing in health and nutrition for over ten years. She wrote her own degree program and graduated in scientific and technical writing from North Dakota State University in 1987 (combination of zoology and journalism). Since then she has written a number of nutrition books. *MSM: Getting Back to Health with Sulfur; PhytoNutrients: Medicinal Nutrients Found in Foods; DHEA: Unlocking the Secrets of the Fountain of Youth—2nd Edition,* co-authored with Richard Ash, M.D., of the Ash Center for Comprehensive Medicine in New York; *How to Fight Osteoporosis and Win! The Miracle of Microcrystalline Hydroxyapatite; The Potato Antioxidant: Alpha Lipoic Acid; Natural Healing Handbook; How Did We Get So Fat?,* coauthored with Dr. Arnold J. Susser of Great Life Labs in Westfield, New Jersey; *Castor Oil: Its Healing Properties;* and *Dr. John Willard on Catalyst Altered Water.* For further information on these books or to order them, please call 1-888-367-3432.

In 1997 she returned to school and recently received her doctoral degree in nutrition.

Dr. Jacobs lives in southern California with her husband, Randy, and two dalmations, Cameo and K.C. She is dedicated to spreading the health message, works out on a regular basis, eats a low-fat vegetarian diet and takes antiaging supplements, including 300 mg of Alpha Lipoic Acid daily.

Memberships: American Academy of Anti-aging, New York Academy of Sciences, Oxygen Society.

WHITAKER WELLNESS INSTITUTE, INC.

is located at

4321 Birch Street
Newport Beach, CA 92660-1923

For more information call:

714-851-1550 or 1-800-283-4584

Index